Short Answer Questions
IN ANAESTHESIA AND CRITICAL CARE MEDICINE

Kingsley Enohumah,
Patrick Olomu,
Charles Imarengiaye

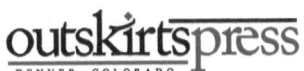
DENVER, COLORADO

The opinions expressed in this manuscript are solely the opinions of the author and do not represent the opinions or thoughts of the publisher. The author has represented and warranted full ownership and/or legal right to publish all the materials in this book.

Short Answer Questions In Anaesthesia And Critical Care Medicine
All Rights Reserved.
Copyright © 2015 Kingsley Enohumah, Patrick Olomu, Charles Imarengiaye
v2.0

This book may not be reproduced, transmitted, or stored in whole or in part by any means, including graphic, electronic, or mechanical without the express written consent of the publisher except in the case of brief quotations embodied in critical articles and reviews.

Outskirts Press, Inc.
http://www.outskirtspress.com

ISBN: 978-1-4787-5958-4

Outskirts Press and the "OP" logo are trademarks belonging to Outskirts Press, Inc.

PRINTED IN THE UNITED STATES OF AMERICA

Dedication

This book is dedicated to our wives and children. Without their support and encouragement this project would have been impossible.

To our teacher Prof. Mathias O. Obiaya, whose light has illuminated our paths.

Contents

Foreword VII

Preface IX

Preparation for the Short Answer Questions (SAQ) 1

Short Answer Questions – Paper 1 3

Short Answer Questions – Paper 2 7

Short Answer Questions – Paper 3 11

Short Answer Questions – Bonus Questions 15

MODEL ANSWERS - Paper 1 17

MODEL ANSWERS - Paper 2 53

MODEL ANSWERS - Paper 3 84

MODEL ANSWERS - Bonus Questions 117

References: 132

INDEX 134

Foreword

The Specialist Anaesthetist can without doubt, claim the title " physician par excellence" as he/she is expected to be knowledgeable of all pathologies (surgical and non-surgical).

The part 1 phase of the Residency Programme, a huddle, though surmountable, requires tremendous hard work both theoretical and practical.

The authors, Specialist Anaesthetists, have not only suggested specimen short answer questions but have supplied acceptable answers. They have extensively covered the many difficult patients' management problems a part 1 candidate is expected to sail through to satisfy the examiners.

However, in order to adequately benefit from this "Vademecum", the candidate (should read/ study Basic Science and Anaesthetic text books in the first instance.

This publication will also be useful to examiners when compiling checklists for short answer questions.

Prof. Sylvia G. Akpan
Internal Assessor
Faculty of Anaesthesia
(NPMCN & FWACS)

Preface

Recently, the West African College of Surgeons (Faculty of Anaesthesia) and the Nigeria postgraduate medical college of Nigeria (Faculty of Anaesthesia) introduced the Short Answer Question format in the Part 1 fellowship examination in Anaesthesia and Critical care medicine. Many candidates, already familiar with the time tested long essay format, may find the concise, time-limited approach of the short essay format quite challenging.

In this book, thirty-four sample Short Answer Questions and model answers are presented. The topics cover the core medical specialties of medicine, surgery, obstetrics and gynaecology, and paediatrics as well as the principles of anaesthetic practice, pain management, intensive care, physics and anaesthetic monitoring. These topics are very likely to be encountered in some form in the examination. Also, the references and the books/journals recommended in this book should serve as an invaluable resource.

Many of the topics have been covered in great detail and we understand that candidates are unlikely to reliably reproduce such detail under examination conditions. Our advise therefore is for the candidate to understand the important concepts of the subject matter and write these in a succinct and logical manner. Candidates should also practice writing timed short answers on other topics not directly covered in this book. This would better prepare you to deliver during the actual examination.

Finally, even though this book is aimed at candidates preparing for the Part 1 Fellowship examination, it should also serve as an indispensable resource for other professional written and oral examinations for candidates around the globe.

K.E
P.O
C.I
2015

Preparation for the Short Answer Questions (SAQ)

What does the SAQ paper consist of?

The Part 1 Fellowship examination consists of two parts –Paper 1 and Paper 11. There are ten (10) main SAQ with two to four subtitles in each part requiring you to write the answers in three hours (3hrs). Each question is allocated 12 marks while each part of the question is allocated marks as indicated in percentages at the end of the question.

How should I prepare?

Do whatever you can in advance to minimise your stress on the day of the examination. Pack your bag the night before and go to bed early. If possible, stay overnight as close to the examination centre as possible. Avoid unnecessary stress of traffic jams and delays on the morning of the examination. Get a good breakfast and something to drink. Empty your bladder before going into the examination hall. Having to leave the examination hall for an urgent bathroom visit is a recipe for disaster and loss of valuable time. You will loose at least 10 minutes of your allotted time; disrupt your thought rhythm, which will seriously disrupt your timing. To avoid this, deal with it before you walk into the examination hall.

Should I use abbreviations and acronyms?

We recommend you write the word in full in the first instance followed by the shorter version in brackets such as Atrial fibrillation (AF). After that, it would be acceptable to use the abbreviation or acronym throughout your answer unless its use is very widespread and common such as INR.

Therefore use abbreviations and acronyms appropriately.

How should I use this book?

You must appreciate that this is not another textbook of anaesthesia. We have structured this book to take a question-oriented approach with an examination-oriented guide.

One of our aims is to enhance your hard work and preparation by introducing methods and systems of answering questions succinctly and accurately.

These techniques are essential to passing your examination and we have carefully included enough detail required to reach a pass standard for each answer. We expect you to use this as a guide to practice writing SAQs prior to sitting the examination.

Recommended reading list

We are only listing these based on experience with the examination questions. It is by no means an exhaustive list.

- The Continuing Education in Anaesthesia, Critical Care and Pain Journal (CEACCP)
- The British Journal of Anaesthesia (BJA). Review articles
- Anaesthesia Tutorial of the Week (ATOTW) is a weekly web-based tutorial hosted by the AAGBI and World Federation of Societies of Anaesthesiologists (WFSA).
- Update in Anaesthesia edition and article archives hosted by the World Federation of Societies of Anaesthesiologists (WFSA)
- Anaesthesia & Intensive Care Medicine journal
- Anaesthesia journal Review articles
- International Journal of obstetric anaesthetists. Review articles
- Your preferred standard anaesthesia textbooks

Short Answer Questions - Content Keyword Breakdown

PAPER 1

Question 1: Obstetric Anaesthesia/ Pre-eclampsia

Question 2: General Anaesthesia – pulmonary function tests/one lung anaesthesia

Question 3: ITU – Mechanical ventilation and Sepsis

Question 4: Anaesthetic complication – Management of intra-operative cardiac arrest

Question 5: General Anaesthesia - Phaeochromocytoma

Question 6: Medicine – Management of Atrial Fibrillation

Question 7: Medicine – Management of Diabetic Ketoacidosis

Question 8: Medicine –Thyroid disease

Question 9: General Anaesthesia – Postoperative nausea and vomiting

Question 10: Emergency medicine/surgery - Management of acute abdomen

PAPER 1
ANSWER ALL QUESTIONS. Three Hour paper
Each question is allocated 12 marks while the marks allocated to each part of the question are indicated in percentages

Question 1
A 26-year-old primigravida presented to the labour ward with a history suggestive of pre-eclampsia
 a. What is pre-eclampsia and how is it diagnosed? (30%)
 b. List the effects of pre-eclampsia on maternal physiology. (20%)
 c. Describe the principles of management of a patient with pre-eclampsia (50%)

Question 2
A 32-year-old male presents with destroyed lung syndrome and is scheduled for a right pneumonectomy:
 a. What tests of pulmonary function are required in this patient? (50%)
 b. What device options are available for achieving one-lung ventilation? (20%)
 c. List the problems of one-lung ventilation? (30%)

Question 3
An 18-year old male was admitted into the intensive care unit following laparotomy and closure of intestinal perforation secondary to typhoid ileitis:
 a. What are the immediate priorities on admission into the ICU? (40%)
 b. How would you wean this patient from the ventilator? (60%)

Question 4
An anaesthetized adult patient is suspected to have suffered from a cardiac arrest intraoperatively.
- a. How would you confirm the diagnosis? (25%)
- b. What ECG rhythms may be seen in this patient? (25%)
- c. How would you manage a refractory shockable rhythm? (50%)

Question 5
Concerning a patient with phaeochromocytoma
a. List the diagnostic criteria for phaeochromocytoma (30%)
b. Outline the preoperative preparation of a patient for adrenalectomy (40%)
c. Describe the intraoperative management for open adrenalectomy (30%)

Question 6
Management of atrial fibrillation:
a. Describe how atrial fibrillation may present. (25%)
b. List causes and risk factors of atrial fibrillation. (25%)
c. What management options are available for atrial fibrillation? (50%)

Question 7
Concerning diabetic ketoacidosis:
- a. List the clinical and biochemical findings that confirm diabetic ketoacidosis (40%)
- b. Outline the management plan for severe diabetic ketoacidosis within the first hour of presentation (60%)

Question 8
A 28-year-old woman presents with toxic goitre.
a. What are the clinical features of thyrotoxicosis? (40%)
b. Outline the investigations for this patient (20%)
c. Outline the treatment of a patient with thyroid storm. (40%)

Question 9
A 33-year-old lady, a non-smoker, with a past history of postoperative nausea and vomiting (PONV) is scheduled for laparoscopic cholecystectomy.
a. List the risk factors for PONV (20%)
b. Outline the basic physiology of nausea and vomiting (20%)
c. Describe the principles underlying the treatment of PONV. (60%)

Question 10
A 60-yearold woman presents with an acute abdomen to the Accident and Emergency Department.
    a. List the differential diagnoses. (40%)
    b. Outline the assessment and investigations that should be done in this patient. (60%)

Short Answer Questions - Content Keyword Breakdown

PAPER 2

Question 1: General Anaesthesia – blood conservation/Jehovah Witness

Question 2: General Anaesthesia – hypertension/geriatric s/ orthopaedic/anaphylaxis

Question 3: General Anaesthesia – Obesity/pain management

Question 4: Medicine/General Anaesthesia- kidney failure / transplantation

Question 5: General Anaesthesia – Trauma and Transport

Question 6: Paediatric Anaesthesia –Down syndrome/ post-tonsillectomy bleeding

Question 7: General Anaesthesia – Management of difficult airway

Question 8: Paediatric Anaesthesia- congenital heart disease

Question 9: Monitoring –Central venous pressure

Question 10: Monitoring – cardiac output measurement

QUESTION PAPERS

PAPER 2

ANSWER ALL QUESTIONS. Three Hour paper
Each question is allocated 12 marks while the marks allocated to each part of the question are indicated in percentages

Question 1
A 57-year-old Jehovah's Witness is scheduled for resection of a colonic tumor in three weeks. Her preoperative haemoglobin is 10.1g/dL.
   a. Enumerate the preoperative preparations for this patient. (40%)
   b. What intraoperative methods may be used to minimize blood transfusion? (60%)

Question 2
An 87-year-old known hypertensive woman with right sub-trochanteric femoral fracture presents for total hip replacement:
   a. How would you investigate this woman for complications of hypertension? (30%)
   b. List the anaesthetic techniques suitable for this procedure. (20%)
   c. What complications are associated with the use of methylmethacrylate and how are they managed? (50%)

Question 3
A 45-year-old obese patient presents for cholecystectomy.
   a. What complications of obesity should be looked for in the preoperative assessment? (50%)
   b. Why is pain management important in this patient? (20%)
   c. What options are available for postoperative pain management? (30%)

Question 4
You are asked to provide anaesthesia for a patient with chronic kidney disease (CKD> stage 4) for kidney transplantation.
   a. What are the organ effects that must be considered? (50%)
   b. Outline the pharmacological factors that must be considered (50%)

Question 5
An adult patient sustained multiple injuries following a motorcycle accident. He is being referred from your secondary healthcare hospital to a tertiary centre for multidisciplinary care:
   a. Enumerate the initial management of this patient (50%)
   b. What preparation should you make before the transfer of this patient? (50%)

Question 6
A 2- year old child with Down syndrome presents for adeno-tonsillectomy:
   a. What are the preoperative anaesthetic considerations? (50%)
   b. Outline the steps you would take in managing post –tonsillectomy bleeding in this child? (50%)

Question 7
Concerning management of the difficult airway:
   a. What predictive tests of difficult airway are available? (40%)
   b. How would you manage a "can't intubate, can't ventilate" situation? (60%)

Question 8
Concerning congenital heart diseases:
   a. How may congenital heart diseases be classified? (30%)
   b. Enumerate the features of a large ventricular septal defect in a 2-year old child. (30%)
   c. How would you investigate this child? (40%)

Question 9
Measurement of central venous pressure:
    a. What are the indications for central venous pressure monitoring? (50%)
    b. List the factors that affect central venous pressure (50%)

Question 10
Measurement of cardiac output:
    a) Enumerate the available methods for cardiac output measurement. (40%)
    b) In what situations will it be indicated? (20%)
    c) Describe one method of measuring cardiac output (40%)

Short Answer Questions - Content Keyword Breakdown

PAPER 3

Question 1: Obstetric anaesthesia/Regional technique

Question 2: Pharmacology – Magnesium sulphate

Question 3: Gynaecology /Regional technique

Question 4: Monitoring –physics / capnography

Question 5: General Anaesthesia – Management of Myasthenia Gravis

Question 6: Paediatric Anaesthesia- Prematurity/pain relief

Question 7: General Anaesthesia – Sickle cell disease

Question 8: Medicine – Management of acute cardiorespiratory decompensation

Question 9: Neuroanaesthesia- ICP

Question 10: Paediatric Anaesthesia- Management of hypertrophic pyloric stenosis

QUESTION PAPERS

PAPER 3

ANSWER ALL QUESTIONS. Three Hour paper
Each question is allocated 12 marks while the marks allocated to each part of the question are indicated in percentages

Question 1
A 24-year-old primigravida is scheduled for an elective caesarean section under combined spinal epidural anaesthesia:
  a. Which dermatomes should be blocked prior to an elective caesarean section and how may adequacy of block be tested? (25%)
  b. How might an initially inadequate block be improved sufficiently to allow surgery to proceed? (25%)
  c. How would you manage the patient if she complains of severe headache postoperatively? (50%)

Question 2
Concerning Magnesium Sulphate:
  a) List the therapeutic uses of magnesium sulphate (50%)
  b) What are the potentially harmful effects of magnesium sulphate? (50%)

Question 3
A 36year old woman with uterine fibroid is scheduled for myomectomy under combined spinal-epidural anaesthesia (CSE).
  a. Describe the technique of CSE (50%)
  b. List the possible complications of the technique (25%)
  c. Describe the management of ONE of the complications (25%)

Question 4
Concerning capnography
   a. Outline the principles of capnography. (25%)
   b. What diagnostic information may be gained from capnography in anaesthetic practice? (50%)
   c. List the clinical situations and locations where continuous capnography should be available. (25%)

Question 5
A 19-year-old female with myasthenia gravis (MG) presents for thymectomy
   a. How is MG diagnosed? (40%)
   b. List the treatment options for patients with MG (20%)
   c. Outline how you would anaesthetise this patient (40%)

Question 6
A 3-month-old premature infant presents for repair of bilateral inguinal hernias and circumcision.
   a. List the anaesthetic concerns in a premature infant (40 %)
   b. Describe the anaesthetic management of this child (40 %)
   c. What options are available for the control of postoperative pain? (20 %)

Question 7
A 20-year-old man with sickle cell anaemia presents for laparoscopic appendicectomy.
   a. Describe the mechanisms of the multi-organ dysfunction caused by sickle cell anaemia (60%)
   b. What are the anaesthetic considerations for sickle cell patients? (40%)

Question 8
A 55-year-old in-patient suddenly collapses in the toilet.
   a. What symptoms and signs might suggest acute pulmonary thromboembolism as a cause of this event? (50%)
   b. List the investigations and characteristic findings that might assist in establishing a diagnosis of pulmonary thromboembolism. (50%).

Question 9
A 60-year-old woman with a meningioma presents for a craniotomy.
   a. How would you evaluate her prior to surgery? (30%)
   b. Describe your anaesthetic management. (40%)
   c. What steps would you take to manage an acute elevation of intracranial pressure during surgery? (30%)

Question 10
A 3-week old neonate presents with suspected hypertrophic pyloric stenosis (HPS)
   a. List the clinical, biochemical, and radiological features of (HPS) (40%)
   b. Outline the preparation of this infant for surgery (30%)
   c. How would you anesthetise this neonate for a laparoscopic pyloromyotomy? (30%)

Short Answer Questions - Content Keyword Breakdown

Bonus Questions

Question 1: Paediatric Anaesthesia- Airway obstruction and management

Question 2: Medicine – Management of acute severe asthma

Question 3: Obstetric anaesthesia- Haemorrhage/massive blood transfusion

Question 4: Medicine- Management of burns in adults patient

Bonus questions

Question 1
A 3-year-old child presents to the Accident and Emergency department with stridor.
  a. List the differential diagnoses of acute stridor in a child (40%)
  b. Outline the management of acute epiglottitis in this child (60%)

Question 2
A 28-year-old female patient is brought to the Accident and Emergency in acute severe asthma.
  a. List the features of acute severe and life-threatening asthma (40%)
  b. Outline your management of this patient (60%)

Question 3
Concerning massive obstetric haemorrhage
  a. What is massive haemorrhage (20%)
  b. List the likely causes of the obstetric haemorrhage? (20%)
  c. Enumerate the principle of treatment of massive obstetric haemorrhage (60%)

Question 4
Concerning adult burns from a house fire
  a. Summarise the assessment of burn depth (50%)
  b. Outline the initial management of this patient within the first 8 hours (50%)

MODEL ANSWERS

Paper 1

Question 1
A 26-year-old primigravida presented to the labour ward with a history suggestive of pre-eclampsia
  a. What is pre-eclampsia and how is it diagnosed? (30%)
  b. List the effects of pre-eclampsia on maternal physiology. (20%)
  c. Describe the principles of management of a patient with pre-eclampsia (50%)

a. What is pre-eclampsia
- Pre-eclampsia is a
  » Multisystem disorder of endothelial dysfunction
  » Characterized by widespread vasoconstriction and increased capillary permeability
  » Gestational proteinuric hypertension developing after 20 weeks gestation.
  » Associated with new-onset proteinuria, resolving after delivery.
- Mild pre-eclampsia is present when there is:
  » Hypertension (SBP 140 mmHg or DBP 90 mmHg)
  » Proteinuria (proteinuria 300 mg/24 hours, or significant increase from baseline)
- Severe pre-eclampsia is when one or more of the following is present:
  » Sustained SBP 160 mmHg or DPB 110 mmHg
  » Evidence of other end-organ damage
  » Deteriorating renal and liver function

- » CNS disturbance (altered vision, headache)
- » Pulmonary oedema
- » Epigastric/right upper quadrant pain
- » Thrombocytopenia
- » HELLP syndrome
- » Evidence of foetal compromise
- » IUGR/Oligohydramnios

REMEMBER THIS MNEMONICS
PPREeclampsia:
Pregnancy **P**roteinuria **R**ising blood pressure **E**dema

- Diagnosis requires:
    - » Pregnancy >20 weeks gestation
    - » Hypertension (diastolic BP >90mmHg or a rise of >15mmHg)
    - » Proteinuria (>300mg/24 hours)
    - » With or without oedema

b. List the effects of pre-eclampsia on maternal physiology.

1. Cardiovascular
    - Low or normal plasma volume
    - Increased systemic vascular resistance (SVR).
    - Increased myocardial contractility
    - Increased or normal cardiac output.
    - Associated increased cardiovascular strain and hyperdynamic left ventricle.
2. Central nervous system
    - Some may be asymptomatic prior to eclampsia.
    - Thrombosis causes micro-infarctions.
    - Hypertensive encephalopathy
    - Cerebral vasospasm.
    - Cerebral haemorrhage/subarachnoid bleed
    - Eclampsia (seizures)
    - Cerebral oedema

- Cortical blindness
- Retinal oedema

3. Renal system
    - Glomerular capillary endotheliosis (capillary endothelial cell engorgement).
    - Renal cortical necrosis
    - Renal tubular necrosis
    - Oliguria and proteinuria.
    - Oedema.

4. Respiratory system
    - Reduced colloid osmotic pressure and damaged vascular endothelium predispose patients t
    - Acute Respiratory Distress Syndrome
    - Pulmonary oedema
    - Laryngeal oedema

5. Hepatic system
    - Subcapsular haematoma and possible periportal necrosis.
    - Liver distension with accompanying pain.
    - HELLP (hypertension, elevated liver enzymes, low platelets) Jaundice

6. Coagulation system
    - Disseminated intravascular coagulation/Fibrin degradation
    - Microangiopathic haemolysis

7. Placenta
    - Placental infarction
    - Placental abruption

8. Foetus
    - Death
    - Preterm birth
    - Intrauterine growth restriction

c. Describe the principles of management of a patient with pre-eclampsia

Management of pre-eclampsia is aimed at eliciting:

Relevant clinical history

- Nulliparity/age of patient/gestational age/new spouse
- Headache of recent onset, right upper quadrant pain
- Decreasing urinary output etc

- Physical Examination:
- General Examination: gravid woman, in the reproductive age bracket, facial puffiness, oedema
- Elevated blood pressure, Uterine size 20weeks and above

- Treatment:

Treatment after diagnosis of pre-eclampsia is aimed at:
- Control of blood pressure
- Fluid management
- Anti-convulsant prophylaxis
- Thromboprophylaxis
- Delivery
- Pain relief in labour (including management of epidural analgesia)
- Anaesthesia for caesarean section delivery and instrumental delivery
- Invasive haemodynamic monitoring as indicated
- Control of blood pressure
- The aim of treatment should be to reduce the blood pressure to not less than 140/90 mm Hg.
- Nifedipine, Hydralazine and Labetolol can all be used.

1. Labetolol (if no asthma)
    - Give 200mg orally. An effect should be seen within 30 minutes. Repeat if necessary after 30 minutes.
    - Commence on 200mg every 8 hours increasing to a maximum dose of 600mg every 6 six hours if necessary.
    - If no effect after 1 hour or where oral treatment is not possible give a bolus of IV Labetolol 50mg and commence a continuous infusion

2. Hydralazine
    - Give a bolus of 5-10mg slowly (over 10-15 minutes) followed by a continuous infusion.
    - Infusion 5–15mg/hr.
    -

3. Nifedipine (second line or if labetolol contraindicated)
    - Give 10mg orally (not slow release) Repeat 6 hourly.

FLUID MANAGEMENT
- Total maintenance fluid intake should not exceed 2.0L/24 hrs.
- Use Hartman's solution at 80 ml/hr.
- Restrict to 1ml/kg per hour
- Hourly urine output; tolerate oliguria 0.25ml/kg per hr.

ANTI-CONVULSANT PROPHYLAXIS
Magnessium Sulphate

- Indicated for treatment of severe pre-eclampsia or eclampsia
- Loading dose of 4g over 15mins and then 1g/hr for 24hrs
- Further 2g bolus if an eclamptic fit occurs.
- Aim for a magnesium level of 2–4mmol/L
- Monitoring of patient on Magnesium Sulphate.
    » Continuous pulse oximetry.
    » Hourly urinary output.

- » Hourly respiratory rate
- » 4 Hourly deep tendon reflexes
- Stop infusion if
  - » Reflexes are absent
  - » Respiratory rate falls below 12/min
  - » Urine output is less than 100 ml in the previous 4 hours.
- Treat magnesium toxicity
  - » Antidote is Calcium Gluconate 10 ml of 10% solution given slowly IV over 2 minutes

Thromboprophylaxis

- Encourage early mobilisation
- All patients should have TED stockings whilst immobile.
- Appropriate anticoagulant

Delivery

- Indications for delivery in pre-eclampsia
  - » Maternal indications
    - Severe, refractory hypertension >24 hours
    - Gestational age of 38 weeks or greater
    - Progressive deterioration of renal /hepatic function
    - Pulmonary oedema
    - Worsening thrombocytopenia, coagulopathy/DIC
    - Eclampsia or progression of neurologic symptoms Suspected placental abruption
    - Persistent severe epigastric pain, nausea, or vomiting
  - » Foetal Indications
    - Foetal distress
    - Severe intrauterine growth restriction
- Adjunctive therapies/ Considerations.
  - » Epidural anaesthesia
  - » Avoid ergometrine/syntometrine in third stage
  - » Obtund pressor response to intubation if GA.
  - » Steroids (betamethasone/dexamethasone) if gestation <34 weeks

Question 2

A 32- year old male presents with destroyed lung syndrome and is scheduled for a right pneumonectomy:
   a. What tests of pulmonary function are required in this patient? (50%)
   b. What device options are available for achieving one-lung ventilation? (20%)
   c. List the problems associated with one-lung ventilation? (30%)

a. What tests of pulmonary function are required in this patient? (50%)

- Detailed assessment of respiratory and cardiovascular function is required to:
    » Identify risks of increased post-operative morbidity and mortality
    » Identify need for post-operative ventilation
    » Determine reversibility of airway obstruction (bronchodilator)
- Focused history and physical examination
    » Nature and extent of disease
    » Cough
    » Dyspnoea
    » Sputum production; less than 25ml/day
- Pulmonary Function Tests (PFTs)
    » Spirometry
    » Other Tests
- Spirometric Tests
    » Forced Vital Capacity (FVC)
        - Normal value is 60 mL/Kg; <15 mL/Kg –inability to cough.
    » Forced Expiratory Volume in 1 second (FEV_1)
        - Preoperative FEV_1 of at least 1.5L needed for pneumonectomy.
        - Predicted postoperative FEV_1 <1.0L –sputum retention.

- Predicted postoperative FEV_1 <0.8L – contraindication to lung resection.
» PFT values are reduced by 20% per lobe – So a right pneumonectomy in this patient will result in a 60% reduction
  - Predicted postoperative FEV1 <40% - poor outcome (consider alternatives to surgery)
» Maximum Breathing Capacity (MBC) – Maximum respiratory rate multiplied by tidal volume over 15 seconds and extrapolated to 1 minute.
  - Normal MBC is 60 -200L/min
  - 25-50L/min- significant respiratory impairment, <25L/min – respiratory cripple.
  - MBC is approximately Peak Expiratory Flow Rate (PEFR) x 0.25 or FEV_1 x 35
» Other Tests
  - Room air Arterial Blood Gas (ABG) – baseline
  - Chest X-ray (hyperinflation, bullae)
  - ECG (Cor Pulmonale from chronic hypoxic vasoconstriction)
  - Echocardiogram (cardiac function)
  - Full Blood Count (leukocytosis – infection)
  - Diffusion Capacity for Carbon Monoxide (DL_{CO}) – parenchymal disease.
  - Flow volume loops
  - Maximum Oxygen consumption <10mL/Kg/min – increased mortality.
  - Cardiac Catheterization and balloon occlusion of pulmonary artery of lung to be resected – Pulmonary Artery Pressure > 25mm Hg, $PaCO_2$ > 45 mm Hg, PaO_2 < 60 mm Hg - poor tolerance of pneumonectomy.

b. What device options are available for achieving one-lung ventilation? (20%)
- Double Lumen Tubes (Right or Left, most reliable and easy conversion to two-lung ventilation)
- Single Lumen tube with integral bronchial blocker (Univent tube)
- Fiberoptic confirmation for optimal placement required

c. List the problems associated with one-lung ventilation? (30%)
- Major problem is Hypoxaemia – caused by:
    - Ventilation perfusion (V/Q) mismatch
    - Lateral decubitus position
- General Anaesthesia with two-lung ventilation causes preferential ventilation of upper (non-dependent) lung coupled with preferential perfusion of lower (dependent) lung – **V/Q mismatch** of lower lung.
- In One Lung Anesthesia
    - No ventilation to upper lung
    - Continued perfusion to upper lung
    - Both result in **shunt** in upper lung
- General Anesthesia attenuates hypoxic pulmonary vasoconstriction which may not reliably decrease shunting.
- Other Problems:
    - Difficulty with lung isolation – difficulty placing DLT or Univent tube
    - Malposition of DLT or Univent tube
    - Blood gas abnormalities – hypercarbia
    - Bronchial rupture and haemorrhage (traumatic placement, cuff overinflation)
    - Problems with lung re-inflation

Question 3

An 18-year-old male was admitted into the intensive care unit following laparotomy and closure of intestinal perforation secondary to typhoid ileitis:

a. What are the immediate priorities on admission into the ICU? (40%)
b. How would you wean this patient from the ventilator? (60%)

a. What are the immediate priorities on admission into the ICU? (40%)

- Ensure airway patency and adequate oxygenation
- Vascular access
- Check any vascular access catheters (arterial, peripheral and central).
- Initial resuscitation (first 6hours)
- Begin resuscitation immediately if hypotensive or lactate > 4mmol/L-Targets will be:
  » CVP 8-12mmHg
  » MAP 65mmHg - norepinephrine or dopamine as first-line vasopressors. Use epinephrine as second-line in norepinephrine/dopamine refractory shock.
  » Urine output 0.5ml/kg/hr
  » Central venous O_2 saturations 70% or mixed venous 65%.
  » Transfusion of packed red cells if Hb 7.0g/dL.
- Ventilation
  » 6ml/kg tidal volumes. Aim for plateau pressure 30cm H_2O.
  » Permissive hypercapnia may be required
- Diagnosis
  » Appropriate blood cultures.
  » No delay in antibiotic administration.
  » Perform imaging studies promptly to confirm positions of ETT and central lines.

- Antibiotic Therapy
    » Begin broad-spectrum antibiotics with good penetration to presumed source and active against likely pathogens as soon as possible, but at least within 1 hour of recognizing sepsis or septic shock.
- Steroids
    » Hydrocortisone < 300mg per day in divided doses can be considered for fluid and vasopressor-refractory shock

On-going care using the mnemonics FASTHUG
- **Feeding** - Ensure appropriate nutritional needs of patient
  Analgesia – Ensure pain and sedation strategy is met
- **Sedation** – Assess sedation daily and consider sedation breaks
- **Thromboprophylaxis** - Give prophylactic dose of subcutaneous low molecular weight heparin unless contraindicated. TED stockings or calf/foot pumps should be applied.
- **Head-up** - Elevate the head of the bed to 30 - 45 degrees to reduce gastro-oesophageal reflux and nosocomial pneumonia in ventilated patients.
- **Ulcer prophylaxis** – Give antacid and mucoprotective agents until enteral feeding is established.
- **Glucose control** - Aim to keep glucose levels 150mg/dL(8- 10mmol/L) using a validated protocol.

Documentation
- Document all of your findings in a systematic way.
- Always clearly date and time your assessment of the patient as well as treatment plan.

Family/next of kin
- Keep family updated with care plan

b. **How would you wean this patient from the ventilator? (60%)**
- Weaning assessment
- Weaning techniques
    » Pressure support ventilation (PSV). Once the PS is at a low level (5–8 cm H_2O), they may be considered for extubation.
    » Synchronized intermittent mandatory ventilation (SIMV). Once a low level has been reached and the patient shows no signs of fatigue, then a trial of PSV/CPAP can be provided
    » Continuing full ventilation with periods of low levels of PSV (5cm H_2O)/CPAP (5 cm H_2O). This is comparable to a T-piece trial.
    » Intermittent trials of spontaneous breathing on at least two occasions a day on a T-piece or CPAP 5 cmH_2O.
    » Once a day spontaneous breathing trial (SBT).
    » Tracheostomy

- Extubation
    » Criteria for extubation:
        - Resolution of the pathology that necessitated IPPV.
        - Adequate arterial oxygenation on a FiO_2 0.5 and PEEP 5 cm H_2O.
        - Haemodynamic stability.
        - Normal acid–base status.
        - Normal fluid and electrolyte status.
        - Adequate protective airway reflexes and ability to cough.
        - Awake and co-operative.
- Bedside tests for likelihood of successful extubation
    » PaO_2/FiO_2 ratio >200 mm Hg (26 kPa)
    » Respiratory rate <35 bpm
    » Tidal volume >5 mL/kg
    » Maximal negative inspiratory pressure 20–30 cm H_2
    » Respiratory rate/tidal volume < 100 min/L

Question 4
An anaesthetised adult patient is suspected to have suffered from a cardiac arrest intra-operatively.
- a. How would you confirm the diagnosis? (25%)
- b. What ECG rhythms may be seen in this patient? (25%)
- c. How would you manage a refractory shockable rhythm? (50%)

a. How would you confirm the diagnosis? (25%)

History – unavailable under anaesthesia but possible risk factors (Goldman Cardiac Risk factors) likely present unless the arrest was anaesthesia induced

- Any precipitating factors (hypoxaemia, exsanguinating hemorrhage, electrolyte and acid-base abnormalities drug overdose)

Physical Examination
- Lifeless appearance
- Absent central pulse (carotid artery)
- Absent or extremely low BP

Monitoring – **continuous ECG monitoring is the most important immediate monitor for the diagnosis of a cardiac arrest in the intra-operative setting.**

Transoesophageal Echocardiogram (TOE) – increasingly being used in the diagnosis of intraoperative arrest and its cause (s)

- Look for (**WHIP**):
    - » **W**all motion abnormalities
    - » **I**schaemia, infarction
    - » **H**ypovolaemia
    - » **P**ericardial tamponade, thrombus

b. **What ECG rhythms may be seen in this patient? (25%)**
    - Ventricular Fibrillation or Pulseless Ventricular Tachycardia (VF/VT) – most common (60%) with best prognosis
    - Asystole (flat line) – 30% of cases
    - Electromechanical dissociation (EMD) or Pulseless Electrical Activity (PEA) – least common with worst prognosis.

c. **How would you manage a refractory shockable rhythm? (50%)**
    Follow recognized evidence based Resuscitation Council (UK) guidance
    Immediate management
    - Confirm cardiac arrest
    - Call for help inform the surgeon and theatre team
    - Perform high quality cardiopulmonary resuscitation (CPR) –appropriate depth, rate (30 compressions: 2 breaths)
    - Call for defibrillator and apply pads on chest – below right clavicle and in V6 position
    - Check rhythm and confirm VF/VT from ECG
    - Continue with chest compression while the appropriate energy is selected on the defibrillator
    - Deliver 1st shock at 150-200J biphasic
    - Resume CPR immediately using 30:2 without rhythm check and continue for 2 minutes
    -

    Refractory VF/VT
    - Pause briefly for Rhythm check and if VF/VT persist, deliver 2nd shock at 150-360J, biphasic
    - Repeat step 5 -6
    - If VF/VT persist deliver 3rd shock at 360J, biphasic
    - Resume chest compression immediately
    - Give Adrenaline 1mg IV and amiodarone 300mg IV while performing a further 2 min CPR
    - Repeat this 2 min CPR-rhythm/pulse check-defibrillation sequence if VF/VT persist
    - Give further adrenaline I mg after alternate shocks (ie every 3-5min)

- Check central pulses and ETCO2 for return of spontaneous cardiac (ROSC) activity
  » If YES – post resuscitation care
  » If NO – continue high quality CPR and change to non-shockable rhythm algorithm

Look for reversible causes (4 Hs and 4 Ts)
I. **H**ypoxia
II. **H**ypovolaemia
III. **H**ypo/hyperkalaemia/metabolic
IV. **H**ypothermia

I. **T**hrombosis - coronary or pulmonary
II. **T**amponade - cardiac
III. **T**oxins
IV. **T**ension pneumothorax

Transoesophageal echocardiogram: Look for cardiac activity, reversible causes.

Question 5
Concerning a patient with phaeochromocytoma
  a. List the diagnostic criteria for phaeochromocytoma (30%)
  b. Outline the preoperative preparation of a patient for adrenalectomy (40%)
  c. Describe the intraoperative management for open adrenalectomy (30%)

a. List the diagnostic criteria for phaeochromocytoma (30%)

A phaeochromocytoma is a catecholamine-secreting tumour arising from the chromaffin cells of the adrenal gland (90%) or other extra adrenal sites (10%).

- History
  » Hypertension (continuous or paroxysmal)
  » Headaches
  » Palpitations
  » Sweating
  » Panic attacks/anxiety
  » Decreased exercise tolerance if myocardial dysfunction is present
  » History of other endocrine neoplasia
- Physical Examination
  » Elevated blood pressure
  » Bradycardia (reflex)
  » Systolic hypertension, diastolic hypotension, and tachycardia if adrenaline is secreted in large amounts
  » Evidence of heart failure or cardiomyopathy
  » Evidence of other endocrine neoplasia
- Investigations
  » Urine
    - Vanillyl mandelic acid (catecholamine metabolite)
    - Homovanillic acid (dopamine metabolite)
  » Blood

- Serum adrenaline, noradrenaline, and dopamine
- Free plasma metanephrine and normetanephrine and 24 hour urine for fractionated metanephrines provide the highest sensitivity and specificity for diagnosis
- Differential venous sampling
» Radiological
    - Nuclear scan: meta-iodobenzyl guanidine (MIBG) scan
    - CT scan
    - MRI, MRA (angiography), MRV (venography)
    - PET scan using fluoro-deoxyglucose F-18
» Pharmacological testing
    - Clonidine suppression test: >40% suppression of plasma metanephrines excludes pheochromocytoma

b. Outline the preoperative preparation of a patient for adrenalectomy (40%)

- Preoperative goals are to:
    » Control hypertension
    » Increase intravascular volume
    » Optimize myocardial function
- Oral anti-hypertensive therapy with non-selective alpha-adrenergic receptor blocking agents (phentolamine or phenoxybenzamine) – up to 2 weeks or more
- Generous oral fluid intake to avoid excessive orthostatic hypotension - Intravenous fluid repletion may be required
- Start beta-adrenergic receptor blocking agent (propranolol) after complete alpha adrenergic blockade (BP and HR within normal range)
    » Severe hypertension, angina, cerebrovascular accident, heart failure and death can occur if started before complete alpha blockade.

- ECG (tachycardia, ventricular hypertrophy)
- Echocardiogram (ventricular hypertrophy, cardiomyopathy, heart failure)
- CXR (cardiomegaly)
- Monitor BP, CVP, Haemoglobin and PAWP (as indicated)
- Withold alpha blockade for at least 12 hours prior to surgery (phenoxybenzamine has a long half-life).
- Administer anxiolytic premedication (midazolam) prior to going to theatre
- Avoid anticholinergics

c. Describe the intraoperative management for open adrenalectomy (30%)

- Intra-operative goals are to:
  » Control sympathetic stimulation from airway management and tumour manipulation
  » Provide cardiovascular support following tumour isolation
- Induction
  » General endotracheal anaesthesia with cardio-stable agents
    - Etomidate, low dose propofol, opiate (fentanyl), muscle relaxant (rocuronium, vecuronium, cis-atracurium)
    - Inhaled agents (sevoflurane, isoflurane)
    - Avoid succinylcholine (fasciculations can cause catecholamines release)
    - Avoid histamine releasing agents (atracurium, succinylcholine, morphine)
    - Avoid halothane (sensitizes myocardium to arrhythmias)
    - Avoid agents that produce vagolysis or sympathetic stimulation (pancuronium, ephedrine, desflurane)

- Monitoring
  » Standard monitoring (BP, HR, SpO$_2$, ECG, E$_T$CO$_2$, Temp).
  » Invasive BP monitoring
  » CVP
  » PAWP as indicated
  » ABGs, Glucose
  » Transoesophageal echocardiogram as indicated.
- Maintenance
  » Inhaled agent and opiates
  » Intravenous fluids
  » Control BP with inhaled agents, sodium nitroprusside, calcium channel blocker (nicardipine), or magnesium sulphate infusion.
  » Esmolol and magnesium sulphate may also be added to antihypertensive regimen
- Post-tumour isolation
  » Dramatic drop in BP occurs: manage as follows:
    - Intravenous fluid loading
    - Vasopressor infusion (noradrenaline, phenylephrine, vasopressin)
  » Monitor for hypoglycaemia
- Role of Epidural analgesia
  » Hypotension may complicate BP control and fluid management
  » Rational approach may be to insert epidural catheter but not use until after cardiovascular stability is achieved post-operatively.
- Transfer to ICU for continuous haemodynamic monitoring

Question 6
Management of atrial fibrillation:
a) Describe how atrial fibrillation may present. (25%)
b) List causes and risk factors of atrial fibrillation. (25%)
c) What management options are available for atrial fibrillation? (50%)

a. Describe how atrial fibrillation may present. (25%)
- » Atrial fibrillation (AF) occurs when there is uncoordinated atrial activity with ventricular rate dependent on AV nodal transmission.
- » It is the commonest cardiac arrhythmia
- » Its incidence increases with advancing age.
- » AF may present as follows:

- Symptoms
  - » Palpitation
  - » Dizziness
  - » Syncope
- Signs:
  - » Irregular pulse or heart beats
  - » No discernible P-wave on ECG
  - » Features of heart failure
  - » Features of systemic embolism

b. List the causes and risk factors for atrial fibrillation. (25%)
- Hypertension
- Rheumatic heart disease
- Ischaemic heart disease
- Congestive heart failure
- Fluid overload
- Cardiomyopathy
- Sick sinus syndrome
- Pulmonary embolism
- Pulmonary hypertension
- Myocarditis

- Hyperthyroidism
- Constrictive heart disease
- Valvular heart disease –mitral valve
- Congenital heart disease (Atrial septal defect)
- Post cardiac surgery
- Diabetes Mellitus
- Respiratory infections
- Neurogenic AF
- Idiopathic
- Familial
- Tobacco use
- Alcohol abuse
- Trauma

c. What management options are available for atrial fibrillation? (50%)

- Goals of treatment
    - Restoration and maintenance of sinus rhythm
    - Control of ventricular response
    - Prevention of thromboembolism
    - Treat any underlying condition
- In acute setting with haemodynamic instability:
    - Synchronized DC cardioversion
        - 200J, 200J, 300J, 360J (monophasic), biphasic with lower current
        - Up to 90% successful
        - Sedation/GA needed
        - Anticoagulation
- In acute setting with haemodynamic stability and AF less than 7 days
    - Pharmacologic cardioversion – Class I and III antiarrhythmics
        - Propafenone, flecainide, ibutilide, dofetilide
        - Amiodarone
        - Anticoagulation
- Maintenance Therapy – maintain sinus rhythm

- » Class I and III antiarrhythmics
- » Class II antiarrhythmics (Sotalol)
- Ventricular rate control
  - » Atrioventricular node conduction blockers
    - Beta blockers (atenolol, metoprolol, esmolol)
    - Digoxin
    - Calcium channel blockers (Verapamil, diltiazem)
- Anticoagulation Therapy
  - » Prior to all cardioversion
    - Heparin
    - Warfarin
  - » Transesophageal echocardiogram to exclude thrombus if anticoagulation is contraindicated
- Non-pharmacologic management
  - » Transvenous atrial pacing
  - » Implantable devices (defibrillator± pacemaker function) Transcatheter ablation
  - » Surgery (Maze procedure)

Question 7
Concerning diabetic ketoacidosis:
a. List the clinical and biochemical findings that confirm diabetic ketoacidosis (40%)
b. Outline the management plan for severe diabetic ketoacidosis within the first hour of presentation (60%)

a. List the clinical and biochemical findings that confirm diabetic ketoacidosis (40%)
- Diabetic Ketoacidosis (DKA) is a serious medical emergency due to insulin deficiency. It is more common in type 1 diabetes and is characterized by hyperglycemia, ketosis, and metabolic acidosis.
- Often precipitated by acute illness such as infection, sepsis
- Mortality is 6-10%

Clinical features
- General
  » Acutely ill looking
  » Dehydration
  » Fever – if acute infection is precipitating factor
- Respiratory
  » Hyperventilation – due to acidosis
  » Ketotic smell in breath – caused by acetone
- Cardiovascular
  » Weak, thready pulse
  » Delayed capillary refill
  » Tachycardia
  » Hypotension
- Gastrointestinal
  » Vomiting
  » Abdominal pain
  » Diarrhoea
- Biochemical findings
  » Severe hyperglycemia >250 mg/dL, serum bicarbonate 18mEq/L, metabolic acidosis on ABG (pH <7.3) and anion gap> 10 mmol are characteristic findings in DKA

- » Full blood count – polycythaemia due to dehydration, leukocytosis from infection
- » Electrolytes
  - hyperkalaemia despite depletion of total body potassium from osmotic diuresis
  - Decreased HCO_3 due to profound acidosis from ketone bodies
  - Anion gap
  - Decreased phosphate and magnesium due to osmotic diuresis
- » Arterial blood gas (ABG) – severe metabolic acidosis
- » Serum osmolality > 300 mOsm/L
- » Elevated beta hydroxybutyrate Hyperamylasaemia, hyperlipasaemia, hypertriglyceridaemia

b. Outline the management plan for severe diabetic ketoacidosis within the first hour of presentation (60%)

Immediate management of DKA (1st hour)
- » Oxygen and airway management as indicated
- » Establish 2 wide bore intravenous lines and start fluid replacement with normal saline (NS) or ½ NS if serum osmolality is >320 mOsm/L
- » Fluid therapy
  - Give 1 L NS in first 30 minutes and then 1 L every hour for the next 2 hours (1.5 L in first hour)
- » Insulin therapy
  - 0.1 units/kg IV bolus followed by:
  - 0.1 units/kg/hour until plasma glucose drops to 180-270 mg/dL (10-15 mmol/L), then 2-4 units/hour thereafter
  - Monitor glucose hourly – goal is to reduce it by 55-90 mg/dL /hour (3-5mmol/L/hour).
- » Insert a central venous line (CVL) – to guide fluid management if indicated
- » Insert arterial line – haemodynamic and blood gas

monitoring
- » Early potassium supplementation is required despite initial hyperkalemia.
  - Give 10-20 mmol in first litre then
  - Give 10-40 mmol per litre depending on plasma potassium levels after first hour
- » Give sodium bicarbonate if pH is < 7.0-7.1 using base excess (BE) as a guide
- » Replace phosphate as potassium phosphate (5-20 mEq) if less than 1.0 mg/dL –over 4 hours.
- » Consider Inserting a nasogastric tube
- Monitoring
  - » Volume status – heart rate, blood pressure, hourly urine output, central venous pressure
  - » Arterial blood gas –hourly
  - » Blood glucose – hourly
  - » Potassium – hourly
  - » Serum osmolality
  - » Ketone stick (ketone bodies in urine)
  - » Sodium, BUN, creatinine – baseline and follow
  - » Phosphate – every 4 -8 hours
  - » Blood/urine culture (sepsis, infection)
  - » CXR
  - » ECG -12 lead and continuous monitoring

Question 8
A 28-year old woman presents with toxic goitre.
   a. What are the clinical features of thyrotoxicosis? (40%)
   b. Outline the investigations for this patient (20%)
   c. Outline the treatment of a patient with thyroid storm. (40%)

a. **What are the clinical features of thyrotoxicosis? (40%)**
   Clinical features of hyperthyroidism/thyroid crisis include:
   - General symptoms
     » Profuse sweating
     » Poor feeding and weight loss
     » Fever and fatigue
   - Cardiovascular
     » Tachycardia, atrial fibrillation, ventricular arrhythmias
     » Heart failure
     » Hypertension (early), hypotension (late)
   - Neurologic
     » Anxiety
     » Tremor and seizure
     » Encephalopathy, coma
     » Weakness and coma
   - Gastrointestinal
     » Diarrhoea, nausea and vomiting
     » Abdominal pains
     » Jaundice
   - Respiratory
     » Dyspnoea
     » Increased oxygen consumption and carbon dioxide production
     » Goitre (possible airway compromise)
     » Reproductive
     » Menstrual disturbances
   - Physical findings
   - Fever
     » Temperature may exceed 38.5 C

- Cardiovascular signs
    - » Hypertension with a wide pulse pressure
    - » Signs of high output heart failure
    - » Hypotension may occur when shock ensues
    - » Tachycardia
    - » Cardiac arrhythmia
- Neurologic signs
    - » May be agitated and confused
    - » Hyperreflexia
    - » Tremor and seizures may occur
    - » Coma
- Others
    - » Sweaty
    - » Orbital signs and goitre as signs of thyrotoxicosis

b. Outline the investigations for this patient (20%)

- FBC
    - » May reveal mild leucocytosis
- Thyroid Function Test (TFT)
    - » The result may not come back quick enough to influence immediate treatment. However usual findings include:
        - elevated triiodothyronine (T3)
        - elevated thyroxine (T4) and free T4 levels
        - increased T3 resin uptake
        - elevated 24-hr iodine uptake
        - suppressed thyroid stimulating hormone (TSH)
- Liver function test and urea and electrolytes
    - » May reveal non specific abnormalities
    - » Hypercalcaemia may occur from thyrotoxicosis
- ABG and urinalysis
    - » To assess and monitor treatment
- Imaging studies
    - » Chest X-Ray
        - May reveal evidence of chest infection
        - May show cardiac enlargement as a result of CCF

- May reveal pulmonary oedema
- May reveal tracheal deviation or compromise in cases of large goiter
- X-ray of neck and thoracic inlet – for mass effect
  » CT scanning
- May help to exclude other neurologic conditions
  » ECG
- Atrial fibrillation is the most common cardiac arrhythmia in thyroid storm
- May also reveal atrial flutter and ventricular tachycardia
- Useful for monitoring these cardiac arrhythmia

c. **Outline the treatment of a patient with thyroid storm. (40%)**
   Treatment is aimed at:
   - **Initial stabilization of patient**
     » Ideally this patient should be managed in the critical care unit
     » Provide supplemental oxygen, airway support and ventilatory support if required
     » Immediate intravenous fluids resuscitation
     » Aggressive control of temperature by
       - Applying ice packs and cooling blankets
       - Administer paracetamol
     » Identify and treat any cardiac arrhythmias and electrolyte abnormalities
   - **Control and relief of hyperadrenergic symptoms**
     » Adrenergic blockade:
       - IV propranolol inhibits peripheral conversion of T4 (thyroxine) to T3 (tri-iodothyronine)
       - Digoxin - controls heart rate and rhythm
       - Amiodarone may inhibit peripheral conversion of T4 to T3 and reduces the concentration of T3-induced adrenoceptors.
   - **Correction of thyroid hormone abnormalities**
     » Propylthiouracil

- Blocks the iodination of tyrosine
- Block peripheral conversion of T4 to T3
- Drug of choice
» Thionamides
- Block the iodination of tyrosine
- Block peripheral conversion of T4 to T3
» Iodines
- Reduces hormonal release from the thyroid
- Enterally administered iodides include
- Lugol's solution
- Sodium or potassium iodide
» Carbimazole
- Only enteral preparations are available
- Metabolised to methimazole
» Methimazole
» Inhibits organification of iodide to iodine and coupling of iodotyrosines
- Lacks peripheral effects
- Only enteral preparations are available
» Glucocorticoids
- Glucocorticoids reduce T4-to-T3 conversion
- Hydrocortisone provides mineralocorticoids activity and glucocorticoid effects
- Dexamethasone provides only the glucocorticoid effects.
- **Supportive measures**
» Fluid management
» Nutrition
- **Other therapy that have been used**
» Plasmapharesis
» Charcoal haemoperfusion
» Dantrolene
- **Investigation and treatment of precipitating factors (e.g. infection)**

Question 9

A 33-year-old lady, a non-smoker, with a past history of postoperative nausea and vomiting (PONV) is now scheduled for a laparoscopic cholecystectomy.

a. List the risk factors for PONV. (20%)
b. Outline the basic physiology of nausea and vomiting. (20%)
c. Describe the principles underlying the treatment of PONV. (60%)

a. List the risk factors for PONV

The risk factors for PONV may be classified as follows:

1. Patient related factors
   - Female gender.
   - Past history of PONV
   - Non-smoker
   - History of motion sickness.
   - Obesity
   - Early ambulation
   - Early postoperative oral intake
2. Surgery related factors
   - Intra-abdominal laparoscopic procedures
   - Duration of surgery (Prolonged surgery)
   - Gastrointestinal surgery.
   - Gynaecological surgery.
   - ENT (blood in stomach), middle ear surgery
   - Extraocular muscle surgery.
   - Intracranial surgery
   - Emergency surgery (full stomach)
3. Anaesthetic related factors
   - Use of intra and post-operative opioids
   - Use of Volatile anaesthetic agents.
   - Use of nitrous oxide
   - Use of anticholinesterases for the reversal of neuromuscular block
   - Etomidate, thiopentone

- High spinal anaesthesia (blocks above T5) Hypotension
- Intra-operative dehydration
- Inexperienced bag and mask ventilation (gastric dilatation)

4. Disease process related
   - Hypoxia
   - Intestinal obstruction
   - Metabolic, e.g. hypoglycaemia
   - Uraemia
5. Miscellaneous factors
   - Fear
   - Excessive pharyngeal manipulation
   - Prolonged fasting
   - Pain

b. **Outline the basic physiology of nausea and vomiting**
   - The central coordinating site for nausea and vomiting is located in the lateral reticular formation in the brainstem
   - The primary control of nausea and vomiting comes from the vomiting centre (VC), which is located in the medulla.
   - The following primary afferent pathways stimulate the VC:
     » The chemoreceptor triggering zone (CRTZ)
     » The vagal mucosal pathway in the gastrointestinal system
     » Neuronal pathways from the vestibular system
     » Reflex afferent pathways from the cerebral cortex and
     » Midbrain afferents.
   - The stimulation of one of the afferent pathways above can activate the VC via:
     » Cholinergic (muscarinic) receptors
     » Histaminergic receptors
     » Serotonergic receptors
     » Dopaminergic receptors
   - The VC receives afferents from the CRTZ located in the

area postrema on the floor of the fourth ventricle
- » These inputs from multiple areas trigger the complex motor response of emesis

c. **Describe the principles underlying the treatment of PONV.**
- The primary focus should be on avoiding or preventing baseline risk factors.

Optimization in the perioperative period
- Avoid or minimise the use of intra and postoperative opioids
- Use of supplemental oxygen perioperatively
- Perioperative intravenous fluid administration

Modification of anaesthetic technique
- Regional anaesthetic should be administered where possible
- Use of propofol based Total Intravenous Anaesthesia (TIVA) if using GA
- Minimise use of neostigmine
- Pharmacological prophylaxis
- This is aimed at targeting the different receptor types linked to the VC
  - » Serotonin (5-HT3) receptors antagonists
- Exert their effects in the CRTZ and at vagal afferents in the gastrointestinal tract.
- Example are ondansetron and granisetron
  - » Dopamine (D2) receptors antagonists.
- Exert their effects in the CRTZ and at vagal afferents in the gastrointestinal tract.
- Examples are droperidol and metoclopramide
  - » Histamine (H1) receptors antagonists.
- Situated mainly in the vestibular labyrinth.
- An example is cyclizine
  - » Cholinergic (muscarinic) receptor antagonists.
- Act in the vestibular labyrinth CRTZ
- Examples are hyoscine, glycopyrrolate, and atropine
  - » Neurokinin-1 (NK-1) receptor antagonist
- Blocks NK-1 receptors in the central and peripheral

- nervous system
    - An example is Aprepitant
        » Corticosteroid
    - Precise mode of action is not well understood
    - May be due to the release of endorphins
    - Endorphins elevate mood and stimulate appetite.
    - An example is dexamethasone
        » Multimodal approach
    - A combination of agents that act on different receptors results in better prophylaxis.
    - An example is 5-HT$_3$ receptor antagonists with droperidol or dexamethasone.
- Non-pharmacologic Prophylaxis
    - Acupuncture/Acupressure
    - Transcutaneous electrical nerve stimulation (TENS)
    - Acupoint stimulation
    - Hypnosis
    - Ginger root

Question 10

A 60-year-old woman presents with an acute abdomen to the Accident and Emergency Department.
  a. List the differential diagnoses. (40%)
  b. Outline your assessment and investigation of this patient (60%)

a. **List the differential diagnoses. (40%)**
- Acute appendicitis
- Acute cholecystitis
- Acute pancreatitis
- Perforated viscus (ulcer, peritonitis)
- Acute diverticulitis
- Acute intestinal ischemia (volvulus, superior mesenteric artery obstruction)
- Acute ureteric colic
- Acute pyelonephritis
- Abdominal aortic aneurysm
- Kidney stones
- Cholelithiasis
- Haemoperitoneum
- Incarcerated/strangulated hernias (abdominal wall, internal hernias)
- Gynaecologic
    » Ovarian masses (torsion, bleeding)
    » Pelvic abscess
    » Tubo-ovarian masses/abscess
- Medical causes
    » Myocardial infarction
    » Diabetic ketoacidosis (DKA)
    » Acute porphyria
    » Adrenal crisis
    » Basilar pneumonia

b. **Outline your assessment and investigation of this patient. (60%)**

History - detailed
- Onset, duration
- Characteristics of pain, location, radiation, aggravating/ameliorating factors
- Associated vomiting, diarrhea, melaena, bloody stool, hematemesis, haematuria, dysuria, fever, cough, angina, hypertension
- Medications

Physical Examination
- General appearance, distressed or not, any diaphoresis, pulse, blood pressure, capillary refill, pallor, chest exam (pneumonia).
- Abdominal examination
  » Tenderness
  » Rebound tenderness
  » Guarding, rigidity (board-like)
  » Tenderness at McBurney's point
  » Elicited signs
    - Rovsing's sign
    - Murphy's sign
    - Cope's sign
    - Psoas sign
    - Straight Leg Raising sign
  » Rectal examination
  » Pelvic examination
- Laboratory and Imaging Tests
  » Full blood count (leucocytosis, anaemia, polycythaemia from dehydration)
  » Urinalysis
  » ECG
  » Occult blood in stool
  » Kidney, Ureter, Bladder (KUB) - Abdominal X-ray to include view of lower chest
    - Sub-diaphragmatic air, dilated bowel loops with

air/fluid levels, abnormal calcifications
  » CXR – basilar pneumonia, pulmonary congestion
- » Computerized Tomography (CT Scan) of abdomen – most complete single test
- » Ultrasound of abdomen (free fluid, blood, gall stones)
- » Trans-vaginal ultrasound as indicated
- » Radionuclide scan -HIDA (hydroxy iminodiacetic acid) scan
- » MRCP (Magnetic Resonance Cholangiopancreatography)
- » ERCP (invasive)
- » Work up myocardial ischaemia/infarction or abdominal aortic aneurysm as indicated.

MODEL ANSWERS

Paper 2

Question 1
A 57-year-old Jehovah's Witness is scheduled for resection of a colonic tumour in three weeks. Her preoperative haemoglobin is 10.1g/dL.
  a. Enumerate the preoperative preparations for this patient. (40%)
  b. What intraoperative methods may be used to minimize blood transfusion? (60%)

a. **Enumerate the preoperative preparations that should be made in this patient. (40%)**
   Pre-operatively
   - **Involve the patient**
     » Discuss with the patient regarding which (if any) blood products they are prepared to accept.
   - **Consultants involvement**
     » Discussion with the surgeon and intensivist
     » Consider Staging the procedure (Limits acute blood loss)
     » Anaesthetic technique (regional anaesthesia eg Combined Spinal Epidural CSE and/or GA)
     » Arrangement for a cell saver system if available and acceptable to patient
     » Requirement for ICU/HDU
   - **Involve a haematologist**
     » Consider pre-op erythropoietin; one bolus 40 000 U or 300U/kg every 3 week

- » Consider pre-op iron; parenteral iron sucrose (Venofer) 200mg x 3 weekly
- » Vitamin B12 and folic acid supplements
- » Adequate protein intake for haemoglobin synthesis
- » Investigate and treat preoperative anaemia
- **Ethical consideration**
  - » Carefully document agreed upon and unacceptable procedures and treatments.

b. What intraoperative methods may be used to minimize blood transfusion? (60%)

Intra-operatively
- » **Anaesthetic considerations**
  - Positioning (avoid venous congestion)
  - Use of local or regional anaesthesia
  - Hypotensive anaesthesia – of proven use but important to weigh risks against benefits
  - Haemodilution techniques–both hypervolaemic and normovolaemic
  - Use of antifibrinolytic agents, e.g. tranexamic acid, aprotinin and desmopressin
  - Use of a cell saver system if available and acceptable to patient

Surgical considerations
- Procedure could be done in stages (Limit acute blood loss)
- Meticulous surgical technique/experienced surgeon
- Balloon occlusion/ligation of arteries that supply the bleeding area

Question 2

An 87-year-old known hypertensive woman with right sub-trochanteric femoral fracture presents for total hip replacement:

a. How would you investigate this woman for complications of hypertension? (30%)
b. List the anaesthetic techniques suitable for this procedure. (20%)
c. What complications are associated with the use of methylmethacrylate and how may they be managed? (50%)

a. How would you investigate this woman for complications of hypertension? (30%)

Hypertension affects virtually every organ system and a thorough preoperative evaluation looking for end organ damage must be undertaken.

- History and Physical Examination
    » Onset, duration, severity, medications
    » Cardiopulmonary: chest pain, angina pectoris, dyspnoea, orthopnoea, palpitations, exercise tolerance, claudication, dizziness, pedal oedema, orthostatic changes in BP, abnormal heart sounds (S3 and S4 Gallop)
    » Central nervous system: Headache, confusion, transient ischemic attacks, cardiovascular accidents, amaurosis, papilloedema and retinopathy.
    » Renal: facial swelling, proteinuria, oedema, oliguria and haematuria.
    » Endocrine: diabetes may be present and complicate hypertension
- Laboratory testing and imaging as indicated by history and physical examination findings.
    » 12-Lead ECG (ischaemic heart disease, left ventricular hypertrophy± strain pattern, conduction abnormalities)
    » Ambulatory ECG (ischaemic heart disease)
    » CXR (left ventricular hypertrophy, left ventricular dilatation, pulmonary congestion, congestive heart

failure)
- » Echocardiogram (chamber enlargement, wall motion abnormalities, diastolic dysfunction, ejection fraction, shortening fraction estimates)
- » Stress Tests (Treadmill, Dipyridamole-thallium scan, stress echocardiogram)
- » Radionuclear imaging
  - Thallium Scan (cold spots are under perfused areas)
  - Technetium Scan (hot spots are under perfused areas)
  - MUGA Scan (Multiple uptake gated acquisition)
  - Dipyridamole-thallium scan
- » Cardiac Catheterization (Gold standard)
- » Doppler study for carotid disease and other peripheral vascular disease.
- » Others: Full Blood Count, Electrolytes, glucose, lipids, BUN, creatinine. Urinalysis (Proteinuria and haematuria)

b. List the anaesthetic techniques suitable for this procedure. (20%)

- Regional techniques
  - » Spinal anaesthesia with intrathecal opioids (fentanyl/morphine/diamorphine)
  - » Epidural anaesthesia
  - » Combined Spinal Epidural (CSE) with intrathecal opioids (fentanyl/morphine/diamorphine)
  - » May add sedation for patient comfort in lateral position
- General anaesthesia (GA) alone with post operative opioid PCA
- Combined Regional and GA
- Peripheral nerve blockade (post operative pain relief)
  - » Femoral nerve, obturator and lateral cutaneous nerve of the thigh block (3-in-1 block)
  - » Psoas compartment block with an infusion catheter

c. **What complications are associated with the use of methylmethacrylate and how may they be managed? (50%)**
- Bone cement implantation syndrome (BCIS) –poorly understood and not uniformly defined.
- BCIS is characterised by
    » Hypoxia, hypotension, or both
    » Unexpected loss of consciousness, around the time of
        - Cementation
        - Prosthesis insertion
        - Reduction of the joint or
        - Limb tourniquet deflation in a patient undergoing cemented bone surgery (occasionally)
    » Hypoxaemia (pulmonary shunting)
    » Pulmonary hypertension (emboli, cement deposition, absorption of volatile monomer)
    » Hypotension (Right ventricular failure is main cause, decreased SVR, dysrhythmias, LV dysfunction)
    » Renal failure from antibiotic-loaded cement
    » Grades:
        - 1- 3 depending on severity of hypoxaemia and hypotension.
        - Grade 3 is cardiovascular collapse requiring CPR.
    » Risk factors:
        - ASA III and >III
        - Pre-existing pulmonary hypertension
        - Significant cardiopulmonary disease
        - Presence of other fractures.
        - Male sex
- Management of BCIS
    » Call for help
    » Inform the surgeon and theatre team
    » Give 100% oxygen
    » Give IV fluids
    » Insert arterial line

- » Consider Inotropes or vasopressor – maintain RV contractility
- » Pulmonary vasodilators
- » Vent hole in distal femur to release pressure
- » If above measures are unsuccessful:
  - Non-invasive CO monitoring
  - Invasive CO monitoring with pulmonary artery catheter
  - Transfer to ICU
- » If in cardiovascular collapse –
  - Activate the cardiac call
  - Consider stopping operation
  - Cover the wound
  - Reposition patient from lateral to supine position
  - Perform CPR
- Prevention of BCIS
  - » Good surgical technique
    - Medullary lavage, good haemostasis before cement insertion
    - Use of a cement gun to enable retrograde cement insertion
    - Venting of the femur
    - Minimising the length of the prosthesis and
    - Minimising the force applied to it during insertion
  - » Good anaesthetic technique
    - Increasing the inspired oxygen concentration at the time of cementation
    - Avoiding intravascular volume depletion
    - Using additional haemodynamic monitoring in high-risk patients
    - Risk stratification – avoid in high risk patients
    - Maintain normovolaemia
    - Aggressive haemodynamic monitoring (CO monitoring, arterial BP)
  - » Avoid bone cement altogether (Non-cemented bone surgery)

Question 3

A 45-year-old obese patient presents for cholecystectomy.

a. What complications of obesity should be looked for in the preoperative assessment? (50%)
b. Why is pain management important in this patient? (20%)
c. What options are available for postoperative pain management? (30%)

a. What complications of obesity should be looked for in the pre-operative? (50%)

Obesity is defined as a Body Mass Index (BMI) of >30 kg/m² and morbid obesity is defined as a BMI ≥40 kg/m². A BMI ≥50 kg/m² is considered super-obesity.

- Respiratory/Airway
  - Obstructive sleep apnea (OSA)
  - Pickwickian syndrome (Obesity Hypoventilation Syndrome)
  - Pulmonary hypertension (increased pulmonary blood volume)
  - Difficult airway (short neck, increased skin folds, redundant soft tissue)
- Cardiovascular
  - Coronary artery disease
  - Right, Left, Biventricular Failure
  - Peripheral Vascular Disease (PVD)
  - Hypertension
  - Atherosclerosis
  - Cardiac arrhythmias
  - Thromboembolism (DVT, varicose veins)
- Gastrointestinal
  - Gallbladder disease
  - GERD (gastroesophageal reflux disease)
  - Fatty liver disease
- Endocrine/Metabolic
  - Diabetes Mellitus/Glucose intolerance
  - Insulin resistance
  - Dyslipidaemia

- » Metabolic syndrome
- » Hypothyroidism
- » Hernias
- Genitourinary
  - » Renal disease
  - » Urinary incontinence
  - » Abnormal uterine bleeding
- Central Nervous system
  - » Pseudotumour cerebri
  - » Strokes
  - » Carpal tunnel syndrome
- Haematological
  - » Hypercoagulable state
  - » Polycythaemia
- Musculoskeletal
  - » Gout
  - » Arthritis
- Skin
  - » Acanthosis nigricans
  - » Difficult venous access
- Mental health
  - » Depression
  - » Social isolation

b. **Why is pain management important in this patient? (20%)**
- Promotes deep breathing
  - » Prevents atelectasis/respiratory complications
- Promotes strong cough
  - » Prevents sputum retention/infection
- Promotes early mobilization
  - » Decreased thromboembolic risks (DVT, Pulmonary embolism)
- Decreased oxygen consumption
- Decreased left ventricular stroke work
- Decreased hospital stay

a. **What options are available for postoperative pain management? (30%)**

Goal is to provide adequate pain control with minimal respiratory depression or sedation

- Regional / Nerve blocks
    » Field block with local anaesthetic infiltration
    » Local wound infusion of local anaesthetic
    » Ultrasound guided nerve blocks – rectus sheath block and transversus abdominis plane (TAP) block
    » Local anaesthetic atomization to gallbladder fossa
- Intravenous agents
    » Cautious opioid boluses (Morphine/pethidine/tramadol)
    » Patient controlled analgesia (morphine)
    » Intravenous paracetamol (acetaminophen)
    » Non-steroidal anti-inflammatory drugs (NSAIDS)
    » Steroids (methylprednisolone)
    » Intravenous anaesthetic adjuvants (lidocaine, ketamine, clonidine, magnesium)

Question 4
You are asked to provide anaesthesia for a patient with chronic kidney disease (CKD> stage 4) for kidney transplantation.
   a. What are the organ effects that should be considered? (50%)
   b. Outline the pharmacological factors that should be considered (50%)

a. **What are the organ effects that should be considered? (50%)**
   The organ effects that should be considered include:
   Cardiovascular system
   - Hypertension
   - Accelerated atherosclerosis
   - Ischaemic heart disease
   - Left ventricular failure
   - Uraemic cardiomyopathy
   - Cerebrovascular accidents
   - Hyperlipidaemias

   Respiratory system
   - Pulmonary oedema
   - Pleural effusions
   - Increased chest infections

   Gastrointestinal system
   - Peptic ulceration
   - Nausea and vomiting

   Musculoskeletal system
   - Osteodystrophy may cause fractures, deformities etc
   - Muscular weakness

   Nervous system
   - Peripheral neuropathies
   - Autonomic neuropathies

   Haematological system
   - Anaemia
   - Increased 2,3-DPG, oxyhaemoglobin dissociation curve shifted to right
   - Decreased platelet count
   - Decreased platelet activity

Mental changes:
- Lassitude, depression
- Psychosis, coma

b. Outline the pharmacological factors that should be considered (50%)

Changes in the pharmacokinetics of drugs in patients with renal failure result from changes in
- Drug protein binding
- Altered drug elimination
- Altered cellular hepatic metabolism

Direct effects
- Toxicity may arise from volatile anaesthetic agents as a result of alteration in renal concentrating capacity induced by fluoride ions.
- Depressant effects of drug metabolites (thiopentone, opioids)

Indirect effects
- All anaesthetics reduce GFR and intraoperative urine flow.
- Alterations in the renin–angiotensin–aldosterone axis, and antidiuretic hormone release.
- Uraemia causes decreased plasma protein binding and CNS depression
- **Intravenous anaesthetic agents**

Thiopental (thiopentone)
- » May cause prolonged anaesthesia because of
  - Depressant effect of uraemia
  - Decreased protein binding
  - Unbound thiopental (thiopentone).

Propofol
- Considered safe in renal failure.
- May cause profound hypotension

Etomidate
- Metabolized in the liver and excreted renally
- Considered safe in renal failure.

Muscle relaxants
Atracurium/*cis*-atracurium/vecuronium/rocuronium
- Considered suitable for this patient as their excretion is independent of the kidney
- Atracurium is broken down by Hofmann degradation thus may be preferred

Pancuronium is best avoided as its action may be prolonged, 80% being eliminated through the kidneys.
Suxamethonium is safe if there is no hyperkalaemia or peripheral neuropathy.

Inhalational agents:
Some volatile agents are degraded to renally excreted metabolites (fluoride ions), which may have toxic effects.

- Sevoflurane and enflurane
  » Are considered safe in renal failure
- Desflurane
  » Has no renal toxicity
- Isoflurane
  » Has low peak fluoride levels and is safe,
- Halothane
  » Is not metabolized to fluoride.
  » May potentiate arrhythmogenic effect

Opioids
Fentanyl /Remifentanil
- Have no active metabolites
- Excretion is mainly by hepatic metabolism

Morphine
- Have active metabolite (morphine-6-glucuronide)
- This may accumulate and cause prolonged effects

Pethidine (Meperidine)
- Have active metabolite (norpethidine)
- This may accumulate and cause toxic effects

Question 5
An adult patient sustained multiple injuries following a motorcycle accident. He is being referred from your secondary healthcare hospital to a tertiary centre for multidisciplinary care:
   a. Enumerate the initial management of this patient (50%)
   b. What preparation would you make before the transfer of this patient? (50%)

a. **Enumerate the initial management of this patient (50%)**
   - Hypoxia and hypovolaemia are the common causes of preventable trauma deaths
   - The initial management of the trauma patient is divided into four phases

Primary survey
   - Airway and cervical spine control
     » Secure definitive airway and stabilize the cervical spine with manual in-line cervical stabilization (MILS) or a rigid cervical collar with lateral blocks
   - Breathing
     » Treat life threatening chest injuries such as
       - Tension pneumothorax
       - Open pneumothorax
       - Flail chest
       - Massive haemothorax
       - Cardiac tamponade
   - Circulation
     » Control any major external haemorrhage
     » Appropriate intravenous access
     » Warm all fluids/blood
   - Disability
     » 1. Assess the size of pupils and their reaction to light.
     » 2. Score the Glasgow Coma Scale (GCS)
   - Exposure/environment
     » Expose the patient with dignity and protect from hypothermia.

- Others
  » If stable take patient for chest, pelvic and full spine X-ray.
  » Consider CT scan as indicated
  » Routine blood investigations (FBC, U&E, ABG, Type and Crossmatch)
  » Tubes- pass urinary catheter and naso/orogastric tubes.

Resuscitation
As in primary survey

Secondary survey
Head-to-toe examination- this should be undertaken when patient's vital signs are relatively stable

Definitive care
Organ support and transfer

b. What preparation would you make before the transfer of this patient? (50%)

Key points to consider when transferring the critically ill are:

Preparation for transport
- Communication with the tertiary centre
- Meticulous patient resuscitation and stabilization
- **Airway**
  » Airway secured and protected
  » C- spine stabilisation
  » Equipment checked
  » Trained and competent transfer personnel
- **Breathing**
  » Patient mechanically ventilated, sedated and paralysed
  » Adequate gas exchange on transport ventilator confirmed by arterial blood gas analysis
  » Adequate oxygen supply on transfer vehicle
  » Stomach decompressed with naso- or orogastric tube
  » SpO_2 monitoring established

- **Circulation**
  - » Adequate intravenous access
  - » Circulating volume optimized
  - » Haemodynamically stable
  - » All lines are patent and secured
  - » Any active bleeding controlled
  - » Long bone/pelvic fractures stabilized
  - » Adequate haemoglobin concentration
- **Disability**
  - » Treat any active seizures
  - » Initial treatments for raised intracranial pressure (if indicated)
  - » Life-threatening electrolyte disturbances corrected
  - » Blood glucose >4 mmol/L
- **Exposure**
  - » Patient adequately covered to prevent heat loss
  - » Temperature monitored

Drugs to carry
- As determined by the transfer needs

Monitoring enroute
- Minimum standard of monitoring as recommended by AAGBI
  - » Continuous presence of appropriately trained staff
  - » ECG
  - » Non-invasive blood pressure
  - » Arterial oxygen saturation (SaO_2)
  - » End tidal carbon dioxide ($ETCO_2$)
  - » Temperature

Mode of transport
- As appropriate and available

Comprehensive handover to receiving hospital

Documentation
- Maintain clear records of all stages of transfer

Question 6

A 2- year old child with Down syndrome presents for adeno-tonsillectomy:
a. What are the preoperative anaesthetic considerations? (50%)
b. Outline the steps you would take in managing post -tonsillectomy bleeding in this child? (50%)

a. What are the preoperative anaesthetic considerations? (50%)

- Down syndrome is the most frequent chromosomal anomaly with an incidence of about 1 in 800 live births. Incidence is increased with maternal age.
- Pre-operative evaluation to identify involvement of organ systems
    - History of congenital heart disease, airway obstruction, Obstructive sleep apnoea (OSA), unstable cervical spine, and hypothyroidism must be elicited.
- Cardiovascular
    - Cardiac defects present in 40-50% of children with Down syndrome
    - Endocardial cushion defects:
        - Atrioventricular canal (AVC)
        - Ventricular Septal Defect (VSD)
        - Atrial Septal Defect (ASD)
        - Patent Ductus Arteriosus (PDA)
        - Tetralogy of Fallot (TOF)
    - Prone to early pulmonary hypertension (cardiac defect, upper airway obstruction)
    - Difficult vascular access
    - ECG, CXR, and Echocardiogram if indicated from history
- Respiratory/Airway
    - Small mouth, large tongue (macroglossia), small jaw (micrognathia)
    - Midface hypoplasia
    - Adenotonsillar hypertrophy
    - Obstructive sleep apnoea (OSA) – polysomnography may be needed

- » Narrow airway (subglottic stenosis)
- Musculo-Skeletal
  - » Short neck
  - » Atlanto-Axial instability (ligamentous laxity, increased anterior atlanto dental interval) – Flexion/extension radiographs or MRI of the cervical spine
  - » Use of MRI scanning of cervical spine increasing
- Central Nervous System
  - » Developmental delay (mental delay)
  - » Hypotonia
- Gastrointestinal
  - » Duodenal stenosis/atresia, Hirschsprung's disease may be associated with Down syndrome
- Endocrine
  - » Hypothyroidism and antithyroid antibodies

b. Outline the steps you would take in managing post –tonsillectomy bleeding in this child? (50%)

- Major concerns for post-tonsillectomy bleeding are:
  - » Hypovolaemia from blood loss and poor oral intake
  - » Anaemia (initial haemoglobin may be deceptively normal –drops with fluid therapy)
  - » "Full stomach" from swallowed blood – increased aspiration and vomiting risks
  - » Bloody and swollen airway – intubation may be technically difficult
- Anaesthetic Management
  - » Start or continue vigorous intravenous fluid resuscitation (20 mL/kg boluses of crystalloid) to include blood transfusion in severe cases (wide bore IV access)
  - » Call for senior help
  - » Focused history and physical examination
    - Pallor, pulse, capillary refill, BP
    - Quickly review anaesthesia record from tonsillectomy
    - Quickly review relevant tests, especially echocardiogram, ECG, any cardiologist's notes

- » Full Blood count, coagulation studies, and type and crossmatch packed cells at time of IV access
- » Prepare theatre
  - Check Anaesthesia machine
  - Two suction setups
  - Multiple cuffed oral RAE tubes with stylet (subglottic stenosis – smaller tube may be needed)
  - ENT surgeon physically present in theatre
  - Rapid sequence induction with cardio-stable agent (ketamine, etomidate), low dose propofol, muscle relaxant (succinylcholine or non-depolarizing agent)
  - Intubate with a styletted cuffed endotracheal tube (smaller size for age in Down syndrome patient)
  - Avoid excessive neck extension for laryngoscopy and by surgeon during surgery.
  - Titrate analgesia – low doses of morpine/fentanyl and IV paracetamol (acetaminophen)
  - Antiemetic (blood in stomach)
  - Have surgeon place gastric tube under direct vision to decompress stomach
  - Respond aggressively to hypotension with crystalloid, colloid, and blood transfusion as indicated
  - Extubate fully awake
  - Transfer to ward or ICU depending on haemodynamics, transfusion, pre-existing cardiac disease.
  - Check post operative haemoglobin

Question 7

Concerning management of the difficult airway:
a. What predictive tests of difficult airway are available? (40%)
b. How would you manage a "can't intubate, can't ventilate" situation? (60%)

a. What predictive tests of difficult airway are available? (40%)

- History
  - Patient age
  - Rheumatoid arthritis
  - Obesity,
  - Syndromes in paediatric patients: Treacher Collins etc
  - acromegaly
  - Head and neck masses/infections/trauma/burns
  - Past history of difficult intubation.
- Physical Examination
  - Airway patency, mouth opening, dentition, palate, prognathism
  - Short neck
  - Interincisor distance <3cm or 2 fingers-breadths.
- Specific Tests
  - Mallampati-Samsoon classification
    - Grading system based on visible structures in the mouth when the mouth is fully opened with the tongue maximally protruded. Head must be in neutral position
    - Class I – hard palate, soft palate, uvula and tonsillar pillars
    - Class II hard palate, soft palate and uvula
    - Class III –hard palate and soft palate
    - Class IV –only hard palate (Samsoon)
  - Thyromental distance (TMD)
- Distance from upper border of the thyroid cartilage to the lower border of the mentum (chin). TMD < 6 cm associated with difficult intubation
- Correlates with cephalad larynx and small mandibular space for the tongue

- Reliability improved when combined with other tests
-

Wilson Risk Score
- Weight, Head and Neck movement, Jaw movement, and receding mandible, Buck teeth.
- Scale of 0-2 for each parameter; maximum score of 10 points
- Score of 4 predicts 90% of difficult intubations

Horizontal length of mandible
- >9 cm is suggestive of a good view on direct laryngoscopy

Mandibulohyoid distance
- Vertical distance between the anterior edge of the hyoid and the mandible on lateral X-ray
- Distance >6 cm suggestive of difficult intubation

Cervical spine movement
- Evaluates atlanto-occipital and atlanto-axial joints
- Flexion and extension views

Prayer sign
- Inability to place both palms flat together
- Indicative of generalised joint disease/immobility

Radiographic studies
- Mostly measurements of lengths, depth, and angles of structures in relation to the mandible and cervical spine
- Ultrasound of the airway
- Computerized Tomography (CT) scans with 3D reconstruction
- MRI of the airway including Cine-MRI
- Combination of indicators improves predictive value.

b. How would you manage a "can't intubate, can't ventilate" situation? (60%)
- A "Can't intubate, Can't ventilate" situation exists when both intubation and facemask ventilation have failed.

- Severe hypoxaemia will occur unless immediate steps are taken to rescue the airway
- Management

Follow Difficult Airway Society (DAS) algorithm (UK).
- Call for help
- Follow Emergency pathway algorithm on Plan D on the DAS guideline
- Proceed immediately to surgical airway access in the neck.
- Perform a cannula or scalpel cricothyroidotomy
- Perform cannula cricothyroidotomy (recommended primary option for anaesthetists)
  » Use wide-bore intravenous cannula or brand name cannula (Patil, Ravussin)
  » Insert through cricothyroid membrane
  » Air aspiration confirms endotracheal placement
  » Attach Jet ventilator and start careful ventilation
  » Confirm lung inflation and exhalation through upper airway
  » Monitor patient for improvement (colour, oxygen saturation, heart rate, BP)
- If above steps are successful with no complications, awaken patient if surgery does not need to proceed.
- If surgery needs to proceed, optimize airway (Retrograde intubation, Aintree catheter)
- If ventilation fails or complications occur (surgical emphysema), convert immediately to surgical cricothyroidotomy (Call ENT or general surgeon)
- Surgical cricothyroidotomy
  » Identify cricothyroid membrane
  » Stab incision and enlarge using scalpel handle, forceps, or dilator
  » Tracheal hook to pull cricoid cartilage inferiorly
  » Insert appropriate size ETT or tracheostomy tube
  » Confirm ETT position (lung inflation, ETCO2)
  » Ventilate with low pressure source

- » Monitor patient for improvement
- » Abandon procedure unless surgery must proceed.
- » Other available equipment for surgical airway access include Quicktrach 1 & 11

Question 8
Classification of congenital heart disease
a. How may congenital heart diseases be classified? (30%)
b. Enumerate the features of a large ventricular septal defect in a 2-year-old child. (30%)
c. How would you investigate this child? (40%)

a. How may congenital heart diseases be classified? (30%)
- 'Simple' left-to-right shunt lesions –cause increased pulmonary blood flow (PBF)
  » Atrial septal defect (ASD)
  » Ventricular septal defect (VSD)
  » Atrioventricular septal defect (AVSD) – also called Atrioventricular Canal (AVC) defect
  » Patent ductus arteriosus (PDA)
  » Aortopulmonary window
- 'Simple' right-to-left shunt lesions – cause decrease in PBF with cyanosis
  » Tetralogy of Fallot [Right ventricular outflow tract obstruction (RVOTO), RV hypertrophy, malaligned VSD, and an overriding aorta]
  » Pulmonary atresia
  » Tricuspid atresia
  » Ebstein's anomaly (downward displacement of tricuspid valve into the RV cavity, atrialization of the RV, malformed RV cavity)
- Complex shunts- cause mixing of PBF and systemic blood
  » Transposition of the great vessels (arteries) (TGV) or (TGA)
  » Truncus Arteriosus
  » Total anomalous pulmonary venous drainage or return (TAPVD) or TAPVR
  » Double outlet right ventricle (DORV)
  » Hypoplastic left heart syndrome (HLHS)
- Obstructive lesions

- » Coarctation of the aorta (CoA)
- » Interrupted aortic arch (IAA)
- » Aortic stenosis
- » Pulmonary stenosis

b. Enumerate the features of a large ventricular septal defect in a 2-year-old child. (30%)

- At age 2 years
  - » The pulmonary vascular resistance (PVR) would have dropped to normal and
  - » A large VSD would therefore cause severe left-to-right shunting, increased pulmonary blood flow relative to systemic flow (Qp/Qs ratio >2:1).
  - » If unchecked/unrepaired, pulmonary vascular occlusive disease (PVOD) will result with a risk of shunt reversal (Eisenmenger complex).

History
- General
  - » Sweating (cardiac failure)
- Rapid breathing caused by:
  - » Increased work of breathing (WOB)
  - » Pulmonary congestion
  - » Increased airway resistance
  - » Decreased pulmonary compliance
- Recurrent pulmonary infections caused by:
  - » Pulmonary venous congestion
- Exercise intolerance caused by:
  - » All of the above
  - » Congestive heart failure (CHF)
- Failure to gain weight caused by:
  - » All of the above

Physical Examination
- General
  - » Small for age
  - » May be cyanosed if shunt reversal has occurred
  - » Pedal oedema if in CHF

- » Finger clubbing
- Cardiovascular
  - » Tachycardia
  - » Hyperactive praecordium
  - » Systolic murmur
  - » P2 heart sound is increased
  - » Loud S2 heart sound if PVOD has occurred
- Respiratory
  - » Tachypnoea
  - » Increased work of breathing (WOB)
  - » Crackles in lung fields
- Abdomen
  - » Hepatomegaly

c. **How would you investigate this child? (40%)**
Investigations
- FBC
  - » May reveal leucocytosis
  - » Anaemia may be present
- CXR
  - » Cardiomegaly (multi-chamber enlargement)
  - » Increased pulmonary vascular markings (congestion, plethora)
  - » Prominent pulmonary arteries
- ECG
  - » Evidence of left ventricular hypertrophy, left atrial hypertrophy, or biventricular hypertrophy
  - » Evidence of right ventricular hypertrophy if PVOD is present
- Echocardiogram
  - » Identifies location (type), size, number and flow pattern across the VSD
  - » Estimates pulmonary artery pressure
  - » Chamber enlargement
  - » Ventricular function
- Cardiac Catheterization

- » The Gold Standard
- Cardiac MRI
  - » Emerging imaging modality

Question 9
Regarding central venous pressure
   a. What are the indications for a central venous catheter insertion? (25%)
   b. What are the indications for central venous pressure monitoring? (25%)
   c. List the factors that affect the central venous pressure (50%)

a. What are the indications for a central venous catheter insertion?
Indications are:
- Difficult peripheral access
- Haemofiltration / haemodialysis/ECM
- Insertion of pacing wires or pulmonary artery catheters.
- Administration of drugs
    » Irritant drugs
    » Long-term treatment (chemotherapy, antibiotics)
    » Long stay patients (e.g. tetanus)
    » Parenteral nutrition
- Haemodynamic monitoring
    » Central venous pressure
    » Mixed/central venous oxygen saturations

b. What are the indications for central venous pressure monitoring? (25%)
- Acute circulatory failure.
- Anticipated massive blood transfusion for fluid replacement therapy.
- Cautious fluid replacement in patients with compromised cardiovascular status.
- Suspected cardiac tamponade
- Fluid resuscitation during goal-directed therapy in severe sepsis

c. **List the factors that affect the central venous pressure (50%)**
   Raised CVP > 10 cm H$_2$O
   - Acute hypervolaemia
   - Congestive cardiac failure
   - RV infarction / ischaemia
   - cor pulmonale, RV failure
   - Pericardial tamponade
   - Constrictive pericarditis, restrictive cardiomyopathy
   - Pulmonary embolus
   - SVC obstruction
   - IPPV
   - Tricuspid incompetence

   Lowered CVP < 3 cmH$_2$O
   - Acute hypovolaemia - haemorrhage
     » GIT / renal losses, burns
   - High output cardiac failure
   - Septicaemia / SIRS
   - Thyrotoxicosis
   - Decreased sympathetic tone - spinal shock, anaphylaxis
     » Spinal / epidural anaesthesia
   - Drugs - vasodilators, histamine release

   Correlation of CVP with LAP

   Poor correlation in the presence of:
   - Impaired LV function, Pulmonary vascular disease / hypertension
   - EF < 40%
   - LV dyskinaesia
   - Myocardial ischaemia
   - LAP > 15 mmHg
   - Right heart disease
   - Severe pulmonary disease, cor pulmonale
   - Acute lung injury

Question 10
Concerning measurement of cardiac output
   a) Enumerate the available methods for cardiac output measurement (40%)
   b) In what situations will it be indicated? (20%)
   c) Describe one method of measuring cardiac output (40%)

a. Enumerate the available methods for cardiac output measurement? (40%)

The different methods of measuring cardiac output (CO) are:
- Pulmonary artery flotation catheter (PAC)
- Oesophageal Doppler monitor (ODM)
  » This is a non-invasive ultrasonic device
  » Measures the velocity of blood flow in the descending thoracic aorta as the frequency of the reflected ultrasound signal changes with flow velocity
- Transoesophageal echocardiography (TOE)
  » Uses Doppler ultrasound.
  » Gives a range of information about ventricular function, wall motion abnormalities and valvular anatomy
  » Very operator dependent
- Pulse contour analysis
  » Examines the arterial waveform
  » Quantifies the stroke volume (SV) and calculates the stroke volume variation (SVV).
  » Used both in LiDCO and PiCC
- Lithium dilution (LiDCO)
  » This is a bolus indicator dilution method of measuring CO.
  » Provides continuous readings of CO, SV and SVV
- Pulse contour CO (PiCCO)
  » Uses a thermodilution technique in conjunction with pulse contour waveform analysis.
  » Cold saline is used
- Produce beat-to-beat determinations of
  » SV, SVV and a continuous measure of CO,

- » Global end-diastolic volume (GEDV),
- » Intrathoracic blood volume (ITBV)
- » Extravascular lung water (EVLW).
- Thoracic electrical bioimpedance
  - » Involves measuring the resistance to current flow through the thorax.
  - » Resistance changes both with the respiratory cycle and with pulsatile blood flow.
  - » These changes allow continuous determination of
    - CO and SV
    - Contractile state and SVR.
- Thermodilution method

b. In what situations will it be indicated? (20%)
- As a diagnostic tool
  - » To assess myocardial function following a cardiac event likely to produce a low output state e.g. myocardial infarct
  - » To assess cardiac function where there may be a high output state e.g. in septic shock
  - » To measure
    - Pulmonary vascular resistances (PVR)
    - Systemic vascular resistances (SVR)
    - Oxygen delivery and consumption
    - Other derivable variables
- As a therapeutic tool
  - » Assist in monitoring the
    - Effects of medical interventions on cardiac output, e.g. colloid or inotropic therapy
    - The efficacy of oxygen delivery

c. **Describe one method of measuring cardiac output (40%)**
   Pulse contour CO (PiCCO)
   - This technique uses a thermodilution technique in conjunction with pulse contour waveform analysis.
   - Cold saline is injected into a central vein and temperature is measured by a thermistor in an arterial cannula located in a large artery (such as the brachial or femoral).
   - The analysed arterial waveform produces beat-to-beat determinations of
     » SV, SVV and a continuous measure of CO
     » Global end-diastolic volume (GEDV)
     » Intrathoracic blood volume (ITBV)
     » Extravascular lung water (EVLW).

MODEL ANSWERS

Paper 3

Question 1
A 24-year-old primivagida is scheduled for an elective caesarean section under combined spinal epidural anaesthesia:
   a. Which dermatomes should be blocked prior to an elective caesarean section and how may adequacy of block be tested? (25%)
   b. How might an initially inadequate block be improved sufficiently to allow surgery to proceed? (25%)
   c. How would you manage the patient if she complains of severe headache postoperatively? (50%)

a. Which dermatomes should be blocked prior to an elective caesarean section and how may adequacy of block be tested? (25%)

- A block from T4 –S 4 is required for a caesarean section even though the principal nerve supply to the uterus is from T10 –T12.
- The uterus is innervated by T10 and the peritoneum has innervations as high as T4.

Testing and documentation of block adequacy is considered a "standard of care"

- Touch < Pinprick < Cold Sensation
- After spinal anaesthesia cutaneous current thresholds have shown:
    » Touch and pressure carried by A beta fibres to recover first
    » Pinprick carried by A delta fibres to recover second
    » Cold carried by C fibres to recover third

Suggested standard include the presence of:
- Loss of light touch from sacral levels to T5 and loss of cold to T4
- Bilateral lower limb motor block

Methods:
- Cold sensation tested using an ethyl chloride spray.
- Ice and alcoholic skin prep may be used as alternatives.
- Gentle pinprick has the advantages of being simple, repeatable, reproducible and applicable. It also allows discrimination between 'sharp' and 'dull' sensation and more closely indicates the level of 'surgical' anaesthesia.
- Bromage test score from 0-4

b. How might an initially inadequate block be improved sufficiently to allow surgery to proceed? (25%)
- Inadequate block is the most common reason for conversion to general anaesthesia, and also a potential source of litigation.
- **If block is inadequate before surgical incision and delivery is not urgent:**
    » Top up with L-Bupivacaine 0.5%- 20ml
    » Other options include:
        - Remove the epidural catheter and perform a subarachnoid block
        - Provide GA
- **If block is inadequate before surgical incision and delivery is urgent**
    » Top up with L-Bupivacaine 0.5%- 20ml plus NaHCO3 8.4%- 2.0ml
    » Or top up with L-Bupivacaine 0.5%- 10ml plus Lidocaine 2% with Adrenaline 1:200,000- 10ml ±NaHCO3 8.4%- 2.0ml
    » Other methods/technique

- Elevate the foot of the bed in the hope that the block will spread upwards
- Remove the epidural catheter and perform a subarachoid block
- Conversion to GA is almost always the best option

Other options include
» Local anaesthetic wound infiltration by surgeon
» IV Ketamine boluses
» Intermittent IV opioid boluses
» Transversus Abdominis Plane (TAP) block and Rectus sheath block intraoperatively

c. How would you manage the patient if she complains of severe headache postoperatively? (50%)

Management of this patient will include
- Relevant History, Physical examination, investigations and treatment
- Relevant History and risk factors evaluation to include:
    » Age of the patient
    » Vaginal delivery
    » Morbid obesity
    » History of headache/migraine prior to procedure
    » Previous history of PDPH
    » Needle shape and side
    » Operator's level of experience
    » Documented difficulty at epidural insertion
    » Epidural insertion technique
    » Onset and duration
        - Headache typically occurs on the 1st or 2nd day after procedure
        - Headache is typically frontal and occipital
        - Worse on ambulating
        - Symptoms may include
            » Neck stiffness
            » Tinnitus
            » Hypacusis

- » Photophobia
- » Nausea and vomiting
- Physical examinations and investigations will be dependent on the clinical findings

Conservative treatment
- Full explanation to the patient, reassurance and detailed documentation in the patient's medical record
- Bed rest
- Adequate fluid hydration
- Simple analgesics (paracetamol and NSAIDS)
- Abdominal binders
- Caffeine - produces cerebral vasoconstriction
- Saline infusion (40-60 mL) reduces the severity of PDPH

Epidural blood patch (EBP)
- Indicated for severe headache or failed conservative management
- Now the definitive treatment of choice
- Two operator technique
- Under aseptic conditions, 15-20 mL of patient's blood obtained by venipuncture and placed immediately into the epidural space, preferably at the level of the puncture by the second operator
- Two separate mechanisms of action of EBP:
  - » Compression of the dural sac raises intracranial pressure, often causing immediate cessation of the headache.
  - » Sealing of the dural leak by the blood clot, so preventing further CSF loss.
- Repeat EBP may be necessary
- Success rate >90% (first procedure) and ~95% if repeated.

Question 2
Concerning Magnesium Sulphate
a) List the therapeutic uses of magnesium sulphate. (50%)
b) What are the potentially harmful effects of magnesium sulphate? (50%)

a. List the indications for the use of magnesium sulphate as a therapeutic agent (50%)

Clinical uses of magnesium sulphate

- Pre-eclampsia and eclampsia
- Tocolysis
- Acute arrhythmias: (e.g. torsade de pointes)
- Hypomagnesaemia
- Tetanus
- Epilepsy
- Subarachnoid haemorrhage.
- Asthma
- Analgesia
- Epidural adjunct to local anaesthetics for postoperative analgesia.
- Constipation and dyspepsia- magnesium is a laxative and an antacid.

b. What are the potentially harmful effects of magnesium sulphate? (50%)

The harmful effects of magnesium sulphate include:

- Central and peripheral nervous systems:
  » Acts as a cerebral vasodilator
  » Depresses the CNS and is sedating
  » Interferes with the release of neurotransmitters at all synaptic junctions
  » Deep tendon reflexes are lost at a blood concentration of 10 mmol
  » Potentiates the action of depolarizing muscle relaxants

- Cardiovascular
  » Produces sympathetic block and inhibition of catecholamine release.
  » Decreases cardiac conduction and diminishes myocardial contractile force.
- Respiratory
  » Reduces bronchomotor tone
  » No effect on respiratory drive
  » Respiratory muscles depression.
- Uterus
  » A powerful tocolytic
  » Crosses the placenta rapidly and may produce hypotonia and apnoea in the newborn.
- Renal
  » Acts as a vasodilator and diuretic
- Magnesium toxicity

Question 3
A 36-year-old woman with uterine fibroid is scheduled for myomectomy under combined spinal-epidural anaesthesia (CSE).
   a. Describe the technique of CSE (50%)
   b. List the possible complications of the technique (25%)
   c. Describe the management of ONE of the complications (25%)

a. **Describe the technique of CSE (50%)**
   - It is an aseptic procedure

Patient assessment:
   - Evaluate the patient for suitability for CSE.
   - Obtain informed consent
   - Monitors attached and baseline values recorded
   - Pre-load with balanced salt solution 10mL/kg

Equipment:
   A check of the CSE tray to include the following:
   - A 25G - 27G atraumatic spinal needle
   - 18G CSE needle or 18G Tuohy needle
   - Multi-orifice epidural catheter with micro filter
   - Sise needle
   - Loss of resistance 10mL syringe
   - Syringes
     » 20ml, 5ml, 2ml syringes

Procedure:
   - Ensure maximum aseptic technique
     » Wear a cap, mask, scrub, gown and glove
   - Patient in sitting or lateral position
   - Sterile preparation; cleaning and drapping
   - L2/3, L3/4 or L4/5 interspace is identified
   - Any one of the above spaces is infiltrated with 2mL of 1% lidocaine
   - A skin puncture is made with the Sise needle
   - The 18G CSE needle is introduced at the chosen interspace to at most 2cm
   - The trocar is removed and Loss of resistance (LOR) syringe

- filled with air or saline is attached
- The needle is advance gently with the knuckle of the non-dominant hand against the patient's back and the dominant hand advance the needle
- LOR to air or saline is checked after each 0.5cm advancement of the needle
- Positive loss of resistance to air is confirmed and the LOR syringe removed
- An appropriate atraumatic needle is passed through the CSE needle into the subarachnoid space
- Reflux of clear CSF, no parasthesiae or blood
- The trocar is removed and heavy 0.5% bupivacaine (2.5 – 3.0mL) is injected
- The epidural catheter is threaded gently to leave 4-5cm in the epidural space
- Epidural needle is withdrawn and catheter taped to skin
- Patient is returned to the supine position
- If doing the 2-needle technique: establish spinal anaesthesia with atraumatic needle and perform epidural block as described above.
- **Note:** that the epidural catheter is untested with both methods!
- Surgery can commence when sensory loss to sensation or pin-prick is at T_4/T_6
- The epidural catheter can be activated once the spinal anaesthesia has receded and surgery has not been completed
- 0.5% bupivacaine is titrated to effect in aliquots of 3-5mL and up to a total of 10-12mL

b. **List the possible complications of the technique (25%)**
   - Hypotension
   - Postdural puncture headache (PDPH)
   - High spinal
   - Total spinal
   - High epidural block
   - Inadequate or patchy block
   - Urinary retention
   - Meningitis
   - Neurological injury
   - Shivering
   - Pruritus

c. **Describe the management of ONE of the complications (25%)**
   - Common complications include:
     » **Hypotension:** physical methods/fluid/vasopressors
     » **Post Dural Puncture Headache (PDPH):** Choice of needle/Fluid/bed rest/simple analgesics/caffeine
     » **Shivering:** Warm drapes/warmed intravenous fluid/pethidine/tramadol etc

   Management of this patient will include
   - Relevant History, Physical examination, investigations and treatment
   - Relevant History and risk factors evaluation to include
     » Age of the patient
     » Vaginal delivery
     » Morbid obesity
     » History of headache/migraine prior to procedure
     » Previous history of PDPH
     » Needle shape and side
     » Operator's level of experience
     » Documented difficulty at epidural insertion
     » Epidural insertion technique
     » Onset and duration
       - Headache typically occurs on the 1st or 2nd day after procedure

- Headache is typically frontal and occipital
- Worse on ambulating
- Symptoms may include
  - Neck stiffness
  - Tinnitus
  - Hypacusis
  - Photophobia
  - Nausea and vomiting
- Physical examinations and investigations will be dependent on the clinical findings

Conservative treatment
- Full explanation to the patient, reassurance and detailed documentation in the patient's medical record
- Bed rest
- Adequate fluid hydration/carbonated drinks/coffee
- Simple analgesics (paracetamol and NSAIDS)
- Abdominal binders
- Caffeine - produces cerebral vasoconstriction
- sumatriptan (serotonin receptor agonist)
- ACTH; exerts its effect by increasing the concentration of beta-endorphin and therefore intravascular volume.
- Saline infusion (40-60 mL) reduces the severity of PDPH

Epidural blood patch (EBP)
- Indicated for severe headache or failed conservative management
- Now the definitive treatment of choice
- Two operator technique
- Under aseptic conditions, 15-20 mL of patient's blood obtained by venipuncture and placed immediately into the epidural space, preferably at the level of the puncture by the second operator
- Two separate mechanisms of action of EBP:
  - Compression of the dural sac raises intracranial pressure, often causing immediate cessation of the headache.

- » Sealing of the dural leak by the blood clot, so preventing further CSF loss.
- Repeat EBP may be necessary
- Success rate >90% (first procedure) and ~95% if repeated.

Question 4
Concerning capnography
a. Outline the principles of capnography. (25%)
b. What diagnostic information can be gained from capnography in anaesthetic practice? (50%)
c. List the clinical situations and locations where continuous capnography should be available. (25%)

a. Outline the principles of capnography (25%)
Capnography is the monitoring of:
- The partial pressure of carbon dioxide (CO_2) concentration in the respiratory gases at the end of expiration (end-tidal) ($ETCO_2$).

The capnometer non-invasively measures
- The CO_2 levels, and gives an $ETCO_2$.
- The normal range for $PaCO_2$ is 35-45 mm Hg.

A capnograph uses the principle of
- Infrared absorption by CO_2.
- CO_2 has a strong absorption band at a wavelength of 4.26μm.
- A CO_2 analyser has three basic components:
  » Infrared radiation source.
  » Infrared photodetector.
  » Two chambers, one for sampling and the other for reference.
- The sampling chamber can either be
  » A main stream analyser (Fast and accurate but increases dead space and weight on the circuit) or
  » A side stream analyser (Light weight).
- The amount of infrared radiation absorbed is proportional to the CO_2 concentration.

Draw a normal capnograph trace with phases of normal waveforms if you can and if time allows.

b. **What diagnostic information may be gained from capnography in anaesthetic practice (50%)**

Adverse respiratory events such as
- Hypoventilation:
    - Oesophageal intubation
        - Circuit disconnections
        - Unsuspected ventilatory failure
- As an aid in diagnosis of:
    - Pulmonary embolism (A sudden drop in end-tidal CO_2 during anaesthesia)
    - circulatory failure and
    - defective breathing circuits
- Monitoring end-tidal CO_2 is useful during cardiopulmonary resuscitation for assessing adequacy of CPR
- Increased $ETCO_2$ as a result of
    - Hypermetabolic states
    - Rebreathing
    - Exhausted CO_2 absorber
    - Increased equipment dead space
    - Reduced tidal volume and respiratory rate.
- Decreased $ETCO_2$ as a result of
    - Hypothermia
    - Reduced cardiac output
    - Hypometabolic states
    - High PEEP
    - Increased respiratory rate and tidal volume
    - Pulmonary embolism

c. **Clinical situations and locations where continuous capnography should be available (25%)**

Continuous capnography should be used in
- All anaesthetised patients, regardless of the airway device used or the location of the patient.
- All patients whose trachea is intubated, regardless of the location of the patient
- All patients undergoing moderate or deep sedation

- All patients undergoing anaesthesia or moderate or deep sedation are recovered
- All patients undergoing advanced life support

Question 5
A 19-year-old female with myasthenia gravis (MG) presents for thymectomy
  a. How is MG diagnosed? (40%)
  b. List the treatment options for patients with MG (20%)
  c. Outline how you would anaesthetise this patient (40%)
  d. How is MG diagnosed? (40%)

Myasthenia gravis (MG) is characterized by skeletal muscle weakness as a result of antibodies targeted at the acetylcholine receptors at the neuromuscular junction. It is the most understood autoimmune disorder.

- History
  » Muscle weakness – worse on exertion and improves with rest
  » Drooping eye lids
  » Bulbar dysfunction (chewing, swallowing difficulties)
  » Pneumonia secondary to aspiration
  » Slurred speech
  » Respiratory difficulty and failure
  » Myasthenic crisis
  » Other auto-immune disorders (rheumatoid arthritis, thyroiditis, or collagen disease)
  » Neonatal MG (antibodies transferred to newborn from mother)
- Physical examination
  » Easy muscle fatigue and weakness
  » Ptosis
  » Overt respiratory failure requiring mechanical ventilation
  » Evidence of bulbar dysfunction
- Diagnostic tests
  » Tensilon (Edrophonium) test – improvement in muscle strength following a small dose
  » Electromyography – fade in strength following repeated stimulation
  » Antibody assay for detection of autoantibodies to

neuromuscular junction acetylcholine receptors
- » Imaging: CT Scan and MRI of the chest for presence of thymoma

b. **List the treatment options for patients with MG (20%)**
- Long-acting anticholinesterase (pyridostigmine 30-180mg every 6 hours)
- Steroid – prednisolone
- Immunosuppresive therapy (azathioprine, cyclophosphamide)
- Intravenous Immune Globulins (IVIG)
- Plasmapheresis
- Surgery (Thymectomy)

c. **Outline how you would anaesthetise this patient (40%)**
- Preoperative evaluation
  - » Evaluate respiratory function and other indicators of poor postoperative function
    - FVC <2.9L
    - MG for 6 or more years
    - Chronic respiratory disease
    - Pyridostigmine dose of 750mg/day
  - » Evaluate aspiration risk
  - » Stop anticholinesterase 4 hours prior to surgery or decrease dose by 20% (observe closely for respiratory compromise) – better slightly myasthenic than cholinergic
  - » Intravenous induction with propofol and an opiate. Avoid non-depolarizing muscle relaxant unless required (no more than 10% of standard dose). Extremely sensitive to non-depolarizing muscle relaxants.
  - » For rapid sequence, apply cricoid pressure. Resistance to succinylcholine (2mg/kg if required)
  - » Careful monitoring of neuromuscular function
  - » Insert a nasogastric tube

- » Establish large bore intravenous access below level of diaphragm (typically on a foot) should superior vena cava be injured/clamped for repair during thymectomy

- » Optimize volume and electrolytes to avoid complicating muscle weakness
- » Allow return of spontaneous respiration (avoids confusion with use of reversal agents – neostigmine, glycopyrrolate).
- » Extubate when strict criteria are met (tidal volume, negative inspiratory force, head lift, forced vital capacity)
- » Have low threshold for post-operative ventilator support until criteria are met.
- » Transfer to ICU or HDU
- » Ensure adequate pain control
- » Chest Physiotherapy
- » Resume enteral pyridostigmine through nasogastric tube in reduced doses and monitor response
- » Multidisciplinary Involvement as indicated – pulmonary medicine, neuromuscular disease, and immunology consultants

Question 6
A 3-month old premature infant presents for repair of bilateral inguinal hernias and circumcision.
   a. List the anaesthetic concerns in a premature infant (40%)
   b. Describe the anaesthetic management of this child (40%)
   c. What options are available for the control of postoperative pain? (20%)

a. List the anesthetic concerns in a premature infant (40%)
An infant born before 37 weeks from the first day of the last menstrual period is considered premature.

- Respiratory system
    » Respiratory distress syndrome (decreased surfactant production)
    » Increased risk of bronchopulmonary dysplasia (BPD)
    » Poor respiratory control with increased risk for apnoea especially with post conceptual age < 60 weeks
    » Increased risk of respiratory failure (decreased type 1 fibers in diaphragm)
- Cardiovascular system
    » Decreased contractile elements in myocardium – limited ability to increase cardiac output
    » Propensity to revert to foetal circulatory patterns
    » Increased risk of right ventricular and biventricular dysfunction
- Renal system
    » Limited ability to retain sodium and bicarbonate
    » Decreased response to aldosterone
    » Increased evaporative water loss
- Central Nervous system
    » Increased pain sensitivity (immature inhibitory pathways)
    » Increased risk of intraventricular hemorrhage and leucomalacia
    » Increased incidence of retinopathy of prematurity (ROP)

- Haematologic system
    - Anaemia of prematurity
    - Decreased oxygen delivery
    - Prone to thrombocytopenia
- Thermoregulation
    - Prone to hypothermia
        - Increased body surface area to weight rati
        - Decreased brown fat stores
        - Non-keratinised skin
        - Decreased non-shivering thermogenesis
    - Higher temperature to maintain thermoneutral environment
- Gastrointestinal/Hepatic
    - Increased risk of necrotising enterocolitis (NEC)
    - Increased incidence of gastroesophageal reflux
    - Prone to hypoglycemia
        - Decreased glycogen stores
        - Decreased gluconeogenesis
    - Immature hepatic function
    - Increased risk of spontaneous, often lethal, hepatic haemorrhage
    - Decreased albumin (increased drug free fraction)

b. **Describe the anaesthetic management of this child (40%)**
- Anaesthetic choices for this patient are:
    - General anaesthesia
    - Regional anaesthesia (subarachnoid, lumbar epidural, or continuous caudal block) – high incidence of failure
    - Combined general and regional techniques
- In view of duration of procedures, combined technique would be most appropriate provided there are no contraindications to a regional technique
- Experienced consultant ± specialist paediatric centre are prerequisites for managing this patient
- Induction of anaesthesia
    - Standard monitors (ECG, NIBP, SpO2)

- » Inhalational induction with sevoflurane if no prior intravenous access
- » Intravenous propofol if IV access present
- » Muscle relaxation with non-depolariser such as cis-atracurium or rocuronium
- » Endotracheal intubation with appropriate size endotracheal tube (2.5-3.5mm) and mechanical ventilation.
- Maintenance of anaesthesia
    - » Sevoflurane/oxygen/air mixture (lowest FIO_2 possible)
    - » Permissive hypercapnia if BPD and compensated respiratory acidosis are present
    - » Analgesia
        - Intravenous acetaminophen 10-15mg/kg
        - Caudal block alone for all procedures– 1mL/kg of 0.125% bupivacaine in 1:200,000 adrenaline– injected through the sacrococcygeal membrane.
        - Bilateral Ilioinguinal and iliohypogastric nerves block by surgeon or ultrasound guided by anaesthetist + penile block
        - Penile block – dorsal penile nerve block and ring block (genital branch of genitofemoral nerve) - using 2-5mL of 0.25% bupivacaine
        - Bilateral Transversus Abdominis Plane (TAP) blocks using ultrasound guidance or landmarks
        - Avoid opiates as much as possible unless plan is for post-operative ventilation
    - » Ventilation strategy: low tidal volume, high rate, PEEP (reduces atelectasis)
    - » Keep warm
    - » Intravenous caffeine 10mg/kg to decrease risk of post-operative apnoea in high risk patients.
    - » Fluids: Lactated ringer's solution at 4mL/kg + any deficits (minimal losses) and 10% Dextrose to maintain normoglycaemia.
- Post-operative
    - » Plan for extubation but have low threshold for

>> postoperative ventilatory support
>> » Apnoea monitoring regardless of anaesthetic technique

c. What options are available for the control of postoperative pain? (20%)

- Blocks as listed above
    - » Caudal block alone
    - » Ilio-inguinal and ilio-hypogastric blocks- by surgeon or ultrasound guided
    - » Penile block (dorsal nerves and genital branch of the genito-femoral nerve)
    - » TAP block
- Intravenous/oral paracetamol (10-15 mg/kg) every 6 hours
- Rectal paracetamol 30mg/kg
- Low dose fentanyl 0.5mcg/kg per dose as indicated for breakthrough pain (increases apnoea risk).

Question 7
A 20-year male with sickle cell anaemia presents for laparoscopic appendicectomy.
a. Describe the mechanisms of the multi-organ dysfunction caused by sickle cell anaemia (60%)
b. What are the anaesthetic considerations for sickle cell patients? (40%)

a. Describe the mechanisms of the multi-organ dysfunction caused sickle cell anaemia (60%)

Sickle cell anaemia is an inherited haemoglobinopathy characterised by chronic haemolytic anaemia and multi-organ damage. It is common in people of African descent, the Mediterranean, Middle East and parts of India.

- Classic teaching: hypoxic conditions cause polymerisation of sickle haemoglobin (HbS).
    » Red cells become sickle shaped, haemolyse and clog microcirculatory vessels
- Current teaching: devastating effects of sickle cell anaemia caused mostly by disruption of nitric oxide (NO) transport from the lungs to vascular endothelium because of the abnormal haemoglobin.
    » Chronic endothelial inflammation
    » Microvascular occlusion
    » End organ vaso-occlusive infarction
- **Systemic involvement in sickle cell anaemia**
    » Haematological
        - Chronic anaemia (6-10g/dL)
        - Multiple transfusions and iron-loading
        - Auto-splenectomy with decreased immune response
    » Pulmonary
        - Pulmonary infarction
        - Acute chest syndrome
        - Pulmonary hypertension
    » Neurologic

- Transient ischaemic attacks
- Strokes
- Meningitis
» Cardiovascular
- Increased cardiac output
- Cardiomegaly
- Cardiomyopathy
» Renal
- Renal medullary infarction
- Decreased renal function
» Musculoskeletal
- Bone pain crisis
- Muscle pain
- Osteomyelitis
- Maxillary overgrowth
- Avascular necrosis
» Gastrointestinal
- Abdominal pain
- Biliary sludging and gall stones
- Hyperbilirubinemia
» Genitourinary
- Haematuria
- Priapism

b. **What are the anaesthetic considerations for sickle cell patients? (40%)**

- Pre-operative
    » Consult haematologist
    » Know baseline/steady state haemoglobin
    » Look for evidence of end organ damage as listed above
    » Determine (in consultation with haematologist) if exchange transfusion would be needed prior to major surgery (aim to achieve haemoglobin S concentration <40%)
    » Avoid preoperative hypoxaemia, hypovolaemia

- (minimise NPO time), acidosis, hypothermia
  - » Prophylactic antibiotics may be required
- Intra-operative
  - » Standard general anaesthetic techniques as appropriate for surgical procedure. In this patient, general endotracheal anaesthesia with intravenous induction, muscle relaxation and opiates
  - » Avoid hypoxia (use high oxygen concentration), hypovolaemia, hypothermia and acidosis
  - » Avoid the use of tourniquets (no Bier Block)
  - » Consider alkalinisation (decreases oxygen affinity thus keeping haemoglobin oxygenated)
- Post-operative
  - » Supplemental oxygen for at least 24 hours
  - » Typically not candidates for same day surgery
  - » Liberal fluid intake
  - » Adequate pain control – Patient controlled analgesia, bolus opiates, non-opiate analgesics, local or regional blocks as appropriate
  - » Incentive Spirometry

Question 8

A 55-year-old in-patient suddenly collapses in the toilet:
  a. What symptoms and signs might suggest acute pulmonary thromboembolism as a cause of this event? (50%)
  b. List the investigations and characteristic findings that might assist in establishing a diagnosis of pulmonary thrombeombolism. (50%).

a. What symptoms and signs might suggest acute pulmonary thromboembolism as a cause of this event? (50%)
- **Symptoms**
  - Dyspnoea and tachypnoea.
- **Physical signs**
  - Sinus tachycardia
  - Hypotension
  - Cool clammy peripheries
  - Confusion.
  - Central and peripheral cyanosis
  - Signs of acute right heart strain:
    - Raised central venous pressure
    - Palpable right ventricular heave
    - Gallop rhythm.
  - Atrial fibrillation due to a dilated right heart.
  - The symptoms and signs described above are not specific to pulmonary embolism; they are often the manifestation of any critical illness

b. List the investigations and characteristic findings that might assist in establishing a diagnosis of pulmonary thromboembolism (50%).

Non-imaging diagnostic methods -
ECG
- ECG is abnormal in over 70% of patients with pulmonary embolism but these changes are nonspecific.
- Common findings are sinus tachycardia and ST segment abnormalities.

- In massive pulmonary embolism, evidence of right heart strain may be seen (right axis deviation, T wave inversion in V1–3). The classic S1-Q3-T3 pattern seldom occurs.
- The ECG is useful in excluding other conditions such as myocardial infarction.

Arterial blood gases
- Changes could be
  » A reduced partial pressure of oxygen in arterial blood (PaO_2)
  » Normal or low partial pressure of carbon dioxide.
  » An abnormal PaO_2 is nonspecific.

Plasma D-dimer enzyme-linked immunosorbent assay (ELISA)
- Although elevated levels of D-dimers are sensitive for the presence of pulmonary embolism they are not specific.

End-Tidal CO_2
- A reduced end-tidal CO_2

Imaging diagnostic methods
  Chest radiography
- Oligaemia in affected areas.
- A wedge-shaped area along the pleural surface.

  Echocardiography
- Transthoracic echocardiography (TTE)
  » Detects right ventricular dilatation and atrial or ventricular
- Transoesophageal echocardiography (TOE).
  » Detects emboli in main and branch pulmonary arteries

Pulmonary angiography
- Remains the gold standard.
- Expensive, invasive, and carries a mortality risk of 0.3%.
- Accurate interpretation dependent on image quality and experience of radiologist

Contrast-enhanced spiral CT
- Emerging as a first-line investigation.
- Faster, less complex, and less operator dependent than angiography.
- Over 90% specificity and sensitivity in diagnosing pulmonary embolism in the main, lobar and segmental pulmonary arteries.

Ventilation–perfusion scanning
- Most common imaging method used in the diagnosis of pulmonary embolism, but it cannot be performed in intubated patients.

Question 9
A 60-year-old woman with a meningioma presents for a craniotomy.
    a. How would you evaluate her prior to surgery? (30%)
    b. Describe your anaesthetic management. (40%)
    c. What steps would you take to manage an acute elevation of intracranial pressure during surgery? (30%)

a. **How would you evaluate her prior to surgery? (30%)**
- History
  - Headaches
  - Evidence of raised intracranial pressure (ICP)
    - Altered mental status
    - Nausea
    - Vomiting
  - Hypertension
  - Visual changes
  - Medications
  - Co-existing disease
- Physical Examination
  - Full neurological examination:
    - Muscle strength and tone
    - Reflexes
    - Cranial nerves function
  - Hypertension
  - Bradycardia
  - Irregular respiration
  - Papilloedema
- Investigations
  - Full blood count
  - Blood chemistry
  - ECG
  - MRI (tumour localisation, midline shift, cerebral oedema)
  - Type and cross-match for packed red blood cells

b. **Describe your anaesthetic management. (40%)**
- Preoperative
    » Review clinical examination and establish baseline neurologic status
    » Establish IV access
    » Light sedation (IV midazolam)
        - Allay anxiety
        - Avoid respiratory depression (hypercapnia can increase ICP)
- Intraoperative
    » AAGBI standard monitors (ECG, SPO_2, NIBP, Temperature)
    » Smooth intravenous induction (lidocaine, fentanyl, propofol, non-depolarizing muscle relaxant) – aim to blunt haemodynamic response to laryngoscopy and intubation
    » Cuffed endotracheal tube 7.5mm
    » Insert arterial line in radial artery
    » Insert second wide bore intravenous access
    » Insert Foley catheter for urinary output
    » Controlled ventilation: maintain mild-moderate hypocapnia
    » Mannitol 0.5-1g/kg to decrease ICP and facilitate surgery
- Maintenance and Emergence
    » Fentanyl / muscle relaxants
    » Low dose inhaled agents in oxygen/air mixture
    » Isotonic crystalloid intravenous fluid (free water can cause cerebral edema)
    » Avoid glucose solution unless for confirmed hypoglycaemia
    » Colloids may be administered for volume repletion
    » Transfuse PRBC for significant blood loss and symptomatic anaemia
    » Extubate carefully to avoid fluctuations in haemodynamic variables and intracranial pressure
        - Assure airway reflexes and minimize haemodynamic response

» Neurologic examination to confirm return to baseline

c. What steps would you take to manage an acute elevation of intracranial pressure during surgery? (30%)
- Maintain arterial oxygenation
- Re-establish deep anaesthesia (avoid straining or coughing against endotracheal tube)
    » Hypnotic/sedative (thiopental, propofol, midazolam, dexmedetomidine)
    » Opiate (fentanyl)
    » Re-dose muscle relaxant
- Elevate head – enhances venous drainage
- Hyperventilate to mild hypocapnia (3.6 - 4kPa), avoid cerebral ischaemia
- Reduce brain water
    » Mannitol (osmotic diuretic) 0.5-1g/kg, requires an intact blood brain barrier (BBB) to prevent rebound cerebral oedema
    » Furosemide (loop diuretic) 5-10mg intravenously and additional doses as indicated
    » Dexamethasone (steroid) 0.5-1.5mg/kg
- Drain CSF with lumbar catheter or intraventricular catheter (if present)
- Other measures
    » Barbiturate coma
    » Hypothermia

Question 10
A 3-week -old neonate presents with suspected hypertrophic pyloric stenosis (HPS)
   a. List the clinical, biochemical, and radiological features of (HPS) (40%)
   b. Outline the preparation of this infant for surgery (30%)
   c. How would you anesthetise this neonate for a laparoscopic pyloromyotomy? (30%)

a. List the clinical, biochemical, and radiological features of (HPS) (40%)

Gastric outlet obstruction caused by muscle hypertrophy at the level of the pylorus. Occurs in 1:500 births, typically presents between 2-6 weeks of age, and mostly in males (80%)

- Clinical
    » Non-bilious projectile vomiting
    » Regurgitation of feeds
    » Jaundice (glucuronyl transferase deficiency)
    » Evidence of dehydration dependent on severity
        - Dry mucous membranes
        - Poor capillary refill
        - Sunken fontanelle
        - Hypotension
        - Oliguria
        - Shock
    » Olive-shaped mass in right hypochondrium
- Biochemical
    » Hypochloraemic, hypokalaemic metabolic alkalosis (loss of gastric hydrochloric acid)
    » Initial renal response is defense of pH: conserves hydrogen ion in exchange for potassium and also dumps bicarbonate.
    » With worsening dehydration, renal response switches to defense of volume: sodium retention in exchange for hydrogen ions and potassium (aldosterone effect) causing

>> worsening hypokalemia and paradoxic aciduria
>> Delayed diagnosis and treatment (rare) presents with severe hypovolaemia/shock and profound metabolic acidosis
- Radiological
  >> Ultrasonography is now the preferred imaging modality to diagnose HPS. Criteria: single wall muscle thickness >3mm, outer wall to outer wall thickness >13mm with pylorus closed.
  >> Barium swallow – now rarely done. Increases risk of aspiration pneumonitis.

b. **Outline the preparation of this infant for surgery (30%)**
- HPS is a medical emergency NOT a surgical emergency. Dehydration and acid-base abnormalities MUST be fully corrected before surgery.
- Nil by mouth and insert nasogastric tube to decompress stomach
- Assess the severity of dehydration
- Replace volume with intravenous Normal Saline in 10-20mL/kg boluses depending on severity of dehydration
- Follow clinical examination for evidence of volume repletion (reversal of above listed clinical features)
- Follow electrolytes, glucose and urine output
- Biochemical parameters that confirm readiness for surgery:
  >> Sodium >135 mmol/L
  >> Chloride >100 mmol/L
  >> Bicarbonate < 30 mmol/L

c. **How would you anaesthetise this neonate for a laparoscopic pyloromyotomy? (30%)**
- Appropriate personnel and facility with experience in specialised paediatric care
- Ensure reliable intravenous access
- Standard monitoring
- Suction stomach in at least 3 quadrants (a fresh orogastric tube is more effective)

- » Pre-oxygenate between position change (commonly desaturate)
- » Suctioning may trigger vomiting
- Rapid sequence induction with cricoid pressure
    - » Appropriate doses of propofol and muscle relaxant (rocuronium)
    - » Endotracheal intubation with 3.0-3.5mm tube and controlled ventilation to maintain normocapnia
- Maintenance
    - » Oxygen/Air/sevoflurane
    - » Analgesia with intravenous acetaminophen 10mg/kg and local anesthetic infiltration
    - » Rectal acetaminophen 30mg/kg
    - » Avoid opiates or other sedatives to decrease risk of post-operative apnea
    - » Maintenance intravenous fluids (normal saline) and dextrose
- Extubate fully awake
- Post-operative monitoring for apnea on ward or HDU

MODEL ANSWERS

Bonus answer Papers

Question 1
A 3-year-old child presents to the Accident and Emergency department with stridor.
    a. List the differential diagnoses of acute stridor in this child (40%)
    b. Outline the management of acute epiglottitis in this child (60%)

a. List the differential diagnoses of acute stridor in this child (50%)
- Epiglottitis
- Croup (laryngotracheobronchitis)
- Airway foreign body
- Retropharyngeal abscess
- Other retropharyngeal collection (haematoma)
- Angioneurotic oedema
- Ludwig's angina
- Giant ranula
- Inhalational injury
- Airway trauma
- Vascular ring with airway compression
- Infectious mononucleosis
- Diphtheria

b. Outline the management of acute epiglottitis in this child (60%)

- Keep child calm (crying may cause complete airway obstruction)
    » Do not upset the child in any way
    » Do not change position
    » Do not separate from parents
    » Do not attempt to start an intravenous line
    » Do not attempt to perform neck X-ray or a CT scan
    » **Absolutely do not attempt airway management in the A&E**
- Give humidified oxygen blow by (do not force mask on child's face)
- Follow departmental guidelines
- Call for senior help
- Call ENT surgeon
- Do not premedicate
- Transfer to theatre
- Prepare equipment for difficult airway management
    » Difficult airway trolley
    » Various blade sizes
    » Various endotracheal tube sizes, bougies, stylets
    » Video laryngoscope
- ENT surgeon in theatre and ready to perform a rigid bronchoscopy and emergent surgical airway
- Apply pulse oximeter
- Perform gentle inhalational induction with 100% oxygen and sevoflurane or halothane
- Apply other monitors (ECG, BP cuff) after child has fallen asleep
- Establish intravenous access
- Perform direct laryngoscopy and intubate when child is under deep inhalational anaesthesia
- Confirm endotracheal placement with capnography
- Send blood for full blood count, chemistry, and blood cultures

- Administer intravenous fluids
- Administer appropriate antibiotic (Haemophilus influenza type B is most common organism)
- Administer intravenous sedation/analgesia
- Place nasogastric tube and administer enteral sedation as needed
- Transfer to PICU
- Can usually be extubated in 24-48 hours after resolution of epiglottic oedema
- Extubate in theatre or PICU: prepare for immediate reintubation

Question 2

A 28-year-old female patient is brought to the Accident and Emergency in acute severe asthma.
 a. List the features of acute severe and life-threatening asthma (40%)
 b. Outline your treatment of this patient (60%)

a. List the features of acute severe and life-threatening asthma (40%)

Asthma is a disease characterized by reversible bronchoconstriction, airway inflammation (oedema) and mucous plugging (secretions

Acute severe asthma is a medical emergency.

Features of Acute severe asthma (any one of these)

- Inability to complete sentence in one breath
- Respiratory rate   25 breaths/min
- Heart rate   110 beats/min
- PEFR 33-50% predicted or best recorded

Features of life-threatening asthma (above features and any one of these)

- PEF <33% best or predicted
- SPO_2 <92%
- PaO2 <8 kPa
- Normal $PaCO_2$ (4.6-6.0 kPa)
- Silent chest
- Cyanosis
- Weak respiration
- Arrhythmias
- Altered mental status (confusion, coma)
- Hypotension
- Near-Fatal Asthma: Raised $PaCO_2$ and/or requiring mechanical ventilation with raised airway pressures

b. **Outline your treatment of this patient (60%)**
   Immediate treatment
   - Rapid evaluation of the airway, breathing and circulation (ABC)
   - Establish intravenous access if not already in place
   - Start a fluid bolus (often hypovolaemic, loosens secretions)
   - Administer oxygen with highest possible FiO_2 to keep SPO_2 at 94-98%
   - Notify senior clinician
   - Pharmacologic treatment – 1st line
     » Nebulised (oxygen driven) Salbutamol 5mg or terbutaline 10mg. Continuous nebulization if poorly responsive.
     » Nebulised (oxygen driven) Ipratropium bromide 0.5mg every 4-6 hours
     » IV hydrocortisone 100mg ± oral prednisolone 40-50mg daily for at least five days or until recovery
     » Do not give any sedatives
   - Chest X-ray if pneumothorax or pneumonia is suspected

   For life threatening asthma
   - Magnesium sulfate 1.2-2g intravenously over 20 minutes following consultation with senior medical staff
   - Continue first line management as above

   Additional management
   - If patient is not improving after 15-30 minutes:
     » Continue nebulised salbutamol as above for life threatening treatment
     » Nebulised ipratropium 0.5 mg every 4-6 hours
     » Consider intravenous salbutamol, terbutaline, or aminophylline
     » Consider subcutaneous, nebulised, intravenous adrenaline
     » Consider intubation and mechanical ventilation
     » Correct fluid and electrolyte abnormalities, especially potassium

- » Transfer to ICU if not already there
- Indications for intubation
  - » Presence of life-threatening features
  - » Worsening blood gases and spirometric tests
- Ventilatory Strategy
  - » Goals are:
    - Provide adequate oxygenation (high FiO_2)
    - Avoid barotrauma (avoid high inflation pressures and PEEP)
    - Allows time to optimize pharmacologic therapy
    - Allow permissive hypercapnia
  - » Strategy
    - Cautious intubation (hypotension and cardiac arrest can occur immediately after intubation) due to hypovolaemia, decreased sympathetic tone, mechanical ventilation
    - Propofol, ketamine, fentanyl, muscle relaxants (non-histamine releasing agents). Avoid morphine and vecuronium (risk of myopathy) as much as possible.
    - Low flow rates
    - Low respiratory rate
    - Prolonged expiratory time (I:E ratio of 1:4) to prevent breath stacking
- Other Adjunctive treatments
  - » Inhalational agents (isoflurane and sevoflurane)
  - » Intravenous ketamine
  - » Antibiotic if evidence of infection is present (fever, purulent sputum, and leucocytosis)
  - » Extra-corporeal membrane oxygenation or for CO_2 clearance
  - » Chest physiotherapy to mobilise secretions

Question 3
Concerning massive obstetric haemorrhage
   a. What is massive haemorrhage (20%)
   b. List the likely causes of the obstetric haemorrhage? (20%)
   c. Enumerate the principle of treatment of massive obstetric haemorrhage (60%)

a. **What is massive obstetric haemorrhage**
   - Massive obstetric haemorrhage is generally regarded as
     » 50% blood volume loss within 3 hours OR
     » Loss of 150ml/min or more
   Alternative definitions are; or :
     » Acute administration of > 10% of Blood Volume in 10 min
     » Acute administration of > 1.5 X the estimated blood volume
     » Replacement of whole BV (Blood Volume) in < 24 hrs
   - Catastrophic Haemorrhage is where blood loss has exceeded two litres, is ongoing **and** there is a clinically obvious coagulopathy
   - **Postpartum haemorrhage (PPH)** is defined as
     » Blood loss of > 500 ml after vaginal delivery, or 1 000 ml post caesarean section.
   - Severe PPH may also be defined as
     » >1 500 ml blood loss
     » At least a 4 U packed cell transfusion
     » A decrease in haemoglobin (Hb) of 4 g/dL, or
     » Any haemorrhage associated with haemodynamic instability.
   - **The "rule of 30" is useful**. This is defined as follows
     » If the haemoglobin (Hb) or haematocrit drops by 30%,
     » The patient's systolic blood pressure drops by 30%
     » The heart rate rises by 30%,
     » The respiratory rate increases to more than 30/minute,
     » Urinary output decreases to <30 mL/hour,
     » The patient is likely to have lost 30% of her blood volume, and is in moderate shock with a potential for severe shock

b. **List the likely causes of obstetric haemorrhage?**
   - The likely causes of obstetric haemorrhage include

The 4Ts
1. Tone (uterine atony or inflammation)
2. Tissue (retained products, placental complications such accreta, increta or percreta)
3. Trauma (cervical and genital tract damage during delivery)
4. Thrombin (coagulation disorder such as DIC, severe pre-eclampsia or HELLP syndrome)
   - Other risk factors include:
     » Prolonged labour
     » Multiple pregnancy
     » Polyhydramnios
     » Large baby
     » Obesity
     » Previous uterine surgery
     » Coagulopathy

c. **Enumerate the principle of treatment of massive obstetric haemorrhage**
   - Early recognition and treatment are essential to ensure the best outcome.
   - **Prompt assessment and immediate resuscitation**
     » Call for additional help immediately
     » Activate the massive obstetric haemorrhage protocol/drill
     » ABCD, 100% oxygen
     » Establish 2 large bore cannulae
     » Request FBC, Coagulation, fibrinogen, U&E and Cross-Match
     » Haemocue, ABG including lactate and Ca^{2+}
     » Fluid resuscitation; or :
       - Crystalloid / colloid 2000mls via rapid infuser or pressure bags e.g. Level 1 ™ Rapid Infuser (can achieve > 500mL/min warmed fluid flow)

- Transfuse blood through fluid warming device.
- Give group specific blood if cross-matched blood not yet available.
- O-negative blood if available and life threatening haemorrhage
- Non-surgical and surgical intervention for uterine atony as discussed below
  - **Medical**
    - "Rub up" the uterus
    - Ergometrine 0.5mg
    - Syntometrine (syntocinon 5 units with ergometrine 500 mcg)
    - Syntocinon 5 units repeated once if necessary
    - Followed by 40units/500mls infusion at 125ml/h
    - Misoprostal /Carboprost (Hemabate or prostaglandin (F_{2a})
  - **Surgical**
    - Delivery of placental
    - B-Lynch suture (brace suture)
    - Uterine tamponade e.g. Rusch urological balloon or Sengstaken-Blakemore tube
    - Surgical ligation of uterine and internal iliac arteries
    - Hysterectomy
    - Compression/clamping aorta to buy time
    - Uterine replacement if uterine inversion
    - Consider interventional radiological procedures (arterial embolisation or balloon occlusion) if available
- Blood warmer and warming blanket/fluid warmer
- Consider preoperative invasive monitoring
- Consider cell salvage if available
- Correct coagulopathy – FFP, cryoprecipitate, platelets
- Consider systemic haemostatic agents
  - Aprotinin (Trasylol®)
  - Vitamin K
  - Tranexamic acid
  - Recombinant Factor VIIa (NovoSeven®)

- Management targets:
  - Hb 8-10g/dL
  - Platelets >75 x 10^9/l
  - PT / APTT ratio < 1.5
  - Fibrinogen >1.0 g/l
  - Ionised Calcium >1mmol/l
  - Lactate < 2 mmol/l
  - Temp >36°C

Use recombinant factor VIIa (Novoseven) when indicated.

- Indications:
  - Patient has received at least one blood-volume exchange transfusion in the last 12 hours and bleeding is continuing.
  - Patient has received 2 pools of Platelets with no demonstrable benefit.
  - Patient has received 1 litre of FFP and/or 10 units of cryoprecipitate with no benefit.
  - Surgical methods to achieve haemostasis have been unsuccessful.

Communication and teamwork
- Allocate roles to team members
- Inform blood transfusion service and haematologist
- Inform portering service for transport of blood samples and collection of blood products

Further Management Plan
- Stand Down/Debriefing
- Detailed documentation in the patient's note
- Transfer to a high dependency unit or intensive care
- Anticipate coagulopathy and treat clinically until coagulation results available

Question 4
Concerning adult burns from a house fire
   a. Summarise the assessment of burn depth (50%)
   b. Initial management of this patient within the first 8 hours (50%)

a. Summarise the assessment of burn depth (50%)
The degree of burn is summarised as follows:
- Erythema (1st degree)
  - Redness
  - Reversible
  - Tissue blanches with pressure
  - Heals within a week
- Superficial partial (2nd degree)
  - Confined to upper third of dermis
  - Blisters, wet pink, painful
  - Tissue blanches with pressure
  - Heals in 10-12 days without scarring
- Deep partial (2nd degree)
  - Involves majority of the inner dermal layer
  - Dry, white, or charred skin
  - Pain is minimal
  - Severe scarring upon healing
  - No tissue blanching with pressure
  - May heal in 2-3 months
- Full thickness (3rd degree)
  - Complete destruction of both layers
  - White, charred, dry
  - Painless
  - Needs to be excised and skin grafted

b. Initial management of this patient within the first 8 hours (50%)

A quick history to ascertain the nature and machanism of the burn and time of burn

Immediate death is the result of coexisting trauma or airway compromise.

- Therefore immediately
    - Call for help
    - Perform a rapid primary survey to assess the status of the patient's
        - Airway, breathing, and circulation, disability, exposure.
        - Quantify the percentage of burn surface area using 'rule of 9'
- The airway
    - Check for signs of upper-airway obstruction and injury
    - Facial or oral burns, singed facial or nasal hair
    - Hoarse voice. Changes in voice suggest laryngeal oedema
    - Carbonaceous sputum or altered mental status suggest the possibility of airway or inhalation injury.
    - Have a low threshold for endotracheal intubation
        - Do not cut the endotracheal tube, as significant facial swelling is likely in the next 24 hours.
    - Consider and treat carbon monoxide poisoning
        - Ventilate with an increased minute volume and 100% oxygen until carboxyhaemaglobin levels are known
    - Consider dexamethasone IV to reduce oedema
- Breathing
    - Assume inhalation injury in any person whose history suggests prolonged entrapment or confinement in an enclosed area of fire.
    - Inhalation injury may include
        - systemic effects of carboxyhaemaglobin (COHb)
        - hydrogen cyanide absorption
        - chemical pneumonitis or a combination of the above .
    - Carbon monoxide poisoning (CMP)
        - CMP is common in house fires
    - Symptoms of CO poisoning are

- headache and malaise (%HbCO level 10–20)
- nausea and vomiting (%HbCO level 30–40) and
- CVS collapse and death (%HbCO level 60–70).

If present, remember that carboxyhaemaglobin (COHb) has a half-life of

- 3-4 hours in room air,
- 30-40 minutes in 100% oxygen and
- 20 minutes in hyperbaric oxygen.
- Therefore consider hyperbaric oxygen therapy in severe cases

Cyanide poisoning (CP)
- This can also be a consequence of a house fire.
- Cyanide is released by burning certain plastics
- CP may cause metabolic acidosis and arterial hypoxaemia.
- Severe cases can be treated with
    » dicobalt edetate, a cyanide chelating agent
    » or with sodium thiosulphate which accelerates cyanide metabolism.

Burns involving the chest or upper airway could also lead to:
- reduced chest wall compliance
- reduced pulmonary compliance
- and reduced Functional Residual Capacity (FRC).
- bronchospasm, bronchorrhoea
- mucous plugging and pulmonary oedema.
- Treatment
    » humidified oxygen
    » bronchodilators and ventilation as necessary.
- Circumferential or deep chest wall burns may restrict breathing
    » Consider escharotomy (incision of the eschar).

Circulation/Fluid therapy
- Start immediate intravenous fluid resuscitation (crystalloid/colloid)
    » in adults with greater than 15% burns
- Establish two wide bore intravenous cannulae or

- intraosseous access
    - Fluid therapy can be calculated using the **Parkland formula**, as follows
        » For the first eight hours give normal maintenance and 2ml/kg per %Body Surface Area over eight hours.
    - Other regime are Mount Vernon formula and Brook formula
    - Monitor fluid resuscitation
        » Urine output should be maintained at 0.5ml/kg/hr.
    - Electrolytes, haematocrit, urine and plasma osmolality
    - Consider blood transfusion if the haemoglobin concentration falls below 8.0g/dL.

Disability
- Look carefully for evidence of head injury
- focal neurology or pupil asymmetry which may suggest neurological injury.
- Monitor patient's
    » blood gas, COHb
    » blood sugar, Electrolytes
    » alcohol level and urine toxicology.

Exposure
- Remove all clothing but avoid hypothermia
- cool the burn with running water or saline
- Cover the patient with dry, sterile sheets or 'cling film'.
- Assess the depth and extent of the burn.
- Debride all bullae and excision of all adherent necrotic tissue

Other considerations
- Hypothermia
    » Measures include
        - keep the room temperature above 30°C and using blood warmers and heating mattresses.
- Infection
    » Topical antimicrobial prophylaxis with flamazine cream and meticulous infection control nursing routines
    » Systemic antibiotics are not used routinely.
    » Administer tetanus immunization as appropriate.

- Nutrition
    - Nasogastric feeding may be necessary.
    - Consider nasojejunal tube
    - A calorie to nitrogen ratio of 100:1 is commonly used.
- Analgesia
    - Regular paracetamol
    - non-steroidal anti-inflammatory drugs (NSAIDs) where not contraindicated
    - Ketamine bolus and Ketamine infusion
    - Titrate intravenous opioid
    - Entonox are useful for dressing changes.
    - Tricyclic antidepressants, such as amitriptyline, can be useful.
- Head up
    - Nurse the patient thirty degrees head up.
- Investigations
    - Full blood count, urea and electrolytes, liver function tests
    - Arterial blood gases with carboxyhaemoglobin levels
    - Coagulation profile
    - Urine analysis
    - Group and save
    - Creatine phosphokinase and urine myoglobin
    - Chest Xray
- Indications for transfer to a specialist centre
    - Full thickness (third degree) burns over 5% BSA
    - Partial thickness (second degree) burns over 10% BSA
    - Any full-thickness or partial-thickness burn involving critical areas (e.g. face, hands, feet, genitals, perineum, skin over any major joint
    - Circumferential burns of the thorax or extremities
    - Significant chemical injury, electrical burns, lightning injury
    - Coexisting major trauma, or presence of significant pre-existing medical conditions
    - Presence of inhalation injury.

References:

1. AAGBI Safety Guideline. Management of Proximal Femoral Fractures 2011. Anaesthesia 2012; 67:85-98
2. Khanna G, Cenovsky J Bone Cement and the implications for anesthesia. Continuing Education in Anaesthesia, Critical Care & pain Vol.12 Number 4, 2012. (pages 213- 216)
3. Foëx P, Sear JW. The surgical Hypertensive patient. Continuing Education in Anaesthesia, Critical Care & Pain. Vol. 4, Number 5, 2004 (pages 139-143)
4. Edwards ND, Reilly CS. Detection of perioperative myocardial ischaemia. BJA 1994;72: 104-115
5. Coté and Lerman's A Practice of Anesthesia for Infants and Children: 5th Edition (2013)
6. Baum VC, O'Flaherty JE. Anesthesia for Genetic, Metabolic, & Dysmorphic Syndromes of Childhood: 2nd Edition
7. Resuscitation Council (UK) Guidelines 2010
8. Ogunnaike BO, Whitten CW. Anesthesia and Obesity. Chapter 47. Clinical Anesthesia by Paul Barash, 6th edition, 2009, 1230-1246
9. Ogunnaike BO, Whitten CW. Evaluation of the Obese Patient. Chapter 23. Anesthesiology by David Longnecker, 2nd edition, 2012, 301-315
10. Rucklidge M, Hinton C. Difficult and failed intubation in Obstetrics. Continuing Education in Anesthesia, Critical Care & Pain Vol. 12 Number 2, 2012 (pages 86-91)
11. Difficult Airway Society (UK) Guidelines (2004)
12. Hagberg CA. Benumof and Hagberg's Airway Management: 3rd Edition 2013
13. Deakin CD. Clinical Notes for the FRCA (1998)
14. Peyton JM, White MC: Anaesthesia for Correction of Congenital Heart Disease (for the specialist or senior trainee) Continuing Education in Anaesthesia, Critical Care & Pain

Vol. 12, Number 1, 2012 (pages 23-27)
15. DiNardo JA. Anesthesia for Cardiac Surgery: 2nd Edition 1997
16. Park MK. Pediatric Cardiology for practitioners: 4th Edition 2002
17. Brunicardi FC. Schwartz's Principles of Surgery: 8th Edition
18. Dudley HAF. Scott: An Aid to Clinical Surgery (International Student Edition): 3rd Edition
19. Bajpai A, Rowland E. Atrial Fibrillation Continuing Education in Anaesthesia, Critical Care & Pain. Vol. 6 Number 6 2006 (pages 219-224
20. Goodwin SR. Sickle cell and Anesthesia. Society for Pediatric Anesthesia Meeting, Winter 2007
21. Reed A, Yudkowitz F. Clinical Cases in Anesthesia: 4th Edition 2014
22. Peiris K, Fell D. The prematurely born infant and anaesthesia. Continuing Education in Anesthesia, Critical Care & Pain Vol. 9, Number 3, 2009 (73-77)

www.ingramcontent.com/pod-product-compliance
Lightning Source LLC
Chambersburg PA
CBHW030757180526
45163CB00003B/1069